D0608124

SUPERCHARGED FOOD

FOR
KIDS

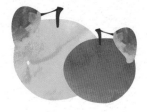

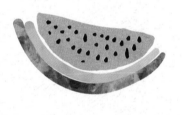

SUPERCHARGED FOOD

FOR
KIDS

Building stronger, healthier, brighter
kids from the ground up

LEE HOLMES

MURDOCH BOOKS
SYDNEY · LONDON

NO LONGER PROPERTY OF
ANYTHINK LIBRARIES/
RANGEVIEW LIBRARY DISTRICT

CONTENTS

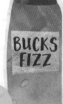
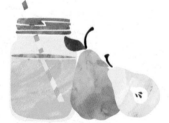
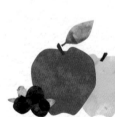

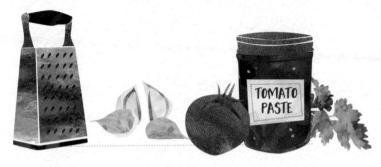

PART TWO RECIPES

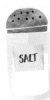

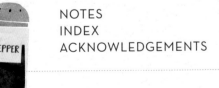

INTRODUCTION

I'm a mum, holistic nutritionist, wholefoods chef and author. As a former English teacher, I've spent a lot of my life in the classroom, helping kids grow academically. Now I want to combine my teaching knowledge with my nutrition and health coaching qualifications to bring you a book that will inspire the whole family to make better food choices. My mission is to change the way children eat so we can build stronger, healthier and brighter kids from the ground up.

This book features meal ideas that not only taste delicious but also deliver the nutrients needed to help kids sustain their energy levels, keep their mood up, concentrate and perform at their best.

Please note: this book is designed to provide general dietary information only for children between the ages of six and twelve. For specific advice on your child's health or dietary and nutritional needs, please contact your GP.

ABOUT THIS BOOK

Getting kids to eat healthily doesn't have to be the Mount Everest of parenthood. In *Supercharged Food for Kids* you'll find recipes that will please even the pickiest of little eaters, plus healthy and delicious options for school lunchboxes, snacks and plenty of dinner ideas that kids will enjoy.

When it comes to school lunches, we always have that niggling feeling that our kids might throw it away and buy something from the canteen instead. Here you'll discover a unique spin on the standard school lunchbox, which too often fails to provide the boost kids need to learn and play throughout the day.

You won't find any Frankenfood (genetically modified food) in *Supercharged Food for Kids*. But you will find kids' favourites, such as pizza, nuggets, pasta and desserts, all made with healthy ingredients. I hope you're inspired to create fresh, wholesome and nutrient-rich meals your children will eat again and again, and to help them develop good eating habits that they can maintain for the rest of their lives.

I also wrote this book to cater for the growing number of children who suffer from food allergies and intolerances, or conditions such as asthma, ADHD, hyperactivity and obesity, or dental problems, digestive issues and learning disorders and difficulties, all of which can be aggravated by poor eating habits. Each recipe is signposted so that you can choose the recipes best suited to your child.

Lee

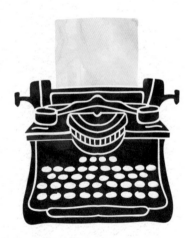

PART ONE

FEEDING HEALTHY, HAPPY KIDS

GETTING STARTED

Whether you're a mum, dad, grandparent or carer (or perhaps a kid yourself), my aim is to inspire you. You'll find an abundance of fun, fast, simple, practical and tasty recipes that won't end up carpeting the floor. I've used good-quality, wholesome foods that encourage healthy eating and snacking but are not puritanical or hard to find in your local supermarket. I believe in the 80/20 rule: try to give your kids healthy options 80 per cent of the time and you're doing well!

To create healthy meals, snacks and lunchboxes for kids, you need to use nutrient-rich wholefoods in a stress-free, practical way. The trick is to keep things as simple as possible. Once you feel comfortable letting the processed and instant foods go, you'll start creating your own meals.

We all know that kids can be the toughest critics, so many of the recipes I've created are healthy versions of familiar favourites, swapping one or two ingredients to make them more nutritious. I've created school sandwiches, wraps, pizza, pasta, nuggets, muffins, energy bars and desserts to appeal to a child's sense of fun and adventure. Even reluctant and picky kids are catered for, with meals that make eating enjoyable without compromising optimum nutrition.

You won't find any low-fat foods here, as their manufacturers often compensate for the loss of fat with large amounts of sugar and additives. I use good fats, which are an essential component of any child's diet, ensuring healthy development and brain function.

When you're making the recipes, wherever feasible, choose foods that are as close to their natural state as possible. This means looking for ingredients that have been produced with the planet in mind, such as organic, fair trade or locally grown or made – where your budget permits. Search for real, unprocessed food.

The serving suggestions are to be used only as a guide, and you can modify the ingredients to suit personal tastes. The recipes also only use equipment that you'll already own. Perhaps best of all is that you can cook up batches of meals and freeze single quantities so they're simple to bring out of the freezer and heat, which really helps if you have a busy schedule.

Included alongside many of the recipes you'll find information about the particular health benefit of the dish; you may also find a Supercharged Tip, which could relate to shopping, storing or cooking.

Once you've read this front section, look through the lunchbox ideas and menus on pages 129–31 and choose some options that suit your family. You can also use these as a guide to create your own meal plan to meet your family's needs. There's a primary shopping list you can work from to make planning easier on pages 45–47.

The World Health Organization's *White Book on Allergy 2011–2012* reports that, worldwide, sensitisation rates to one or more common allergens among schoolchildren are currently approaching 40–50 per cent. In other words, almost half of all children have a food allergy or intolerance of some kind. As you work your way through this book, you'll notice at-a-glance icons that indicate whether the recipe is suitable for children with allergies and intolerances.

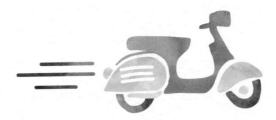

YOUR CHILD'S NUTRIENT NEEDS

The need for nutrient-dense wholefoods for children has never been greater. If you've previously used RDIs (recommended daily intakes) to meet your child's nutritional needs, then think again. The RDIs are general guidelines aimed at the prevention of disease, not the optimisation of health. The RDI for vitamin C, for example, is based on the amount that is known to prevent scurvy.

The nutritional requirements of children are immense, and their needs per unit of weight are much higher than those of adults due to their astounding growth rates. Children require larger amounts of protein for growth than for maintenance, whereas adults use most of their protein intake for maintenance only. A child's liver holds approximately four hours of reserve glucose, so they need to eat in small, frequent bursts to stabilise their blood sugar.

I asked Sydney-based paediatric nutritionist and naturopath Emma Sutherland, who treats children of all ages, to outline the most important nutrients children need for growth and development.

✳ **ZINC** is crucial as a structural component of growing cells and it provides the framework for cells to function at their best. Zinc will increase immunity and help balance blood sugar levels. It's important to note that children low in zinc have a higher incidence of food allergies. Zinc can be found in grass-fed beef and lamb, sesame seeds, pepitas (pumpkin seeds), egg yolk and brazil nuts.

✳ **IRON** is vital for oxygen circulation, keeps the immune system healthy and helps produce energy. Dietary iron comes in two forms: haem iron (found in meat) and non-haem iron (found in plant foods). Iron-rich foods include grass-fed red meat, lentils, asparagus, spinach, egg yolks, blackstrap molasses, raw cacao and spirulina. Note that excessive dairy consumption can reduce iron absorption.

✦ **CALCIUM** requirements for children are high, especially between birth and puberty, when a child's bone structure increases sevenfold. Aim for your kids to get at least 1000 mg per day, as calcium is vital for muscle function as well as strong bones. If you give dairy products to your child, ensure they're full-fat and certified organic, if possible. Or if your child has a dairy allergy or intolerance, give them calcium-rich alternatives, such as sardines, almonds, unhulled sesame seeds, flaxseed, parsley, broccoli, spinach, watercress and figs. Note that vitamin D is important for calcification of bone, so make sure your child runs around in the sun at a low-UV time of day.

✦ **MAGNESIUM** is the most relaxing mineral of all and crucial for growing children. It helps build strong bones and balance blood sugar. A magnesium deficiency can cause irritability, restlessness, poor sleep and muscle cramps. Research has shown a tendency for overweight children to be lower in magnesium. This can easily be addressed by giving them magnesium-rich foods such as pepitas, sunflower seeds, spinach, sesame seeds, cashews, almonds, raw cacao, and sea vegetables such as dulse and kelp.

 SUPERCHARGED TIP A comforting drink can be made by blending 40 g (1½ oz/¼ cup) sunflower seeds with 250 ml (9 fl oz/1 cup) warm water and serving with a touch of raw cacao and vanilla powder.

✦ **OMEGA-3 ESSENTIAL FATTY ACIDS** are vital for the nervous system, and a deficiency can result in impaired learning and behavioural changes. Omega-3s reduce inflammation, making them invaluable for sufferers of eczema, asthma and hayfever. Aim to eat oily fish such as salmon, ocean trout, mackerel and sardines twice a week, and add flaxseed meal and walnuts to meals.

 SUPERCHARGED TIP Sprinkle flaxseed meal in a smoothie or throw some walnuts into your muffin recipe.

✷ **PROTEIN** provides building blocks for growth and development as well as forming the basis of antibodies to help boost immunity. Children low in protein are more susceptible to infections and experience more sugar and salt cravings. Ensure your child has regular protein from a variety of sources, such as grass-fed meat, organic poultry (including turkey), oily fish, nuts, seeds, legumes, lentils and spirulina.

✷ **B VITAMINS** help growing bodies unlock the energy found in fats, proteins and carbohydrates. They're water-soluble and therefore required in small, frequent doses throughout the day. Good sources of B vitamins include grass-fed meat, organic poultry, salmon, eggs, dark-green leafy vegetables, mushrooms, organic liver and spirulina.

✷ **VITAMIN C** is a critical nutrient for growing bodies, as it is a potent antioxidant, increases iron absorption and boosts immunity. Vitamin C plays an important structural role in the formation of collagen and therefore aids wound healing. Foods high in vitamin C include papaya, red capsicum (pepper), strawberries, blackcurrants, oranges, broccoli, pineapples, kiwifruit and goji berries.

 SUPERCHARGED TIP Add dulse flakes to wet dishes such as soups, casseroles and salad dressings to increase iodine levels, which are notoriously low in children.

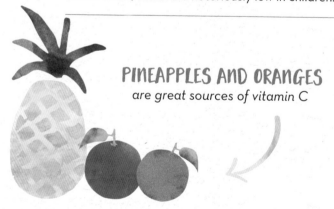

PINEAPPLES AND ORANGES
are great sources of vitamin C

FOOD ALLERGIES AND INTOLERANCES

Rates of allergies and food intolerances among our children are skyrocketing. But what's the difference between a food allergy and a food intolerance?

FOOD ALLERGIES

A food allergy occurs when the immune system reacts to a particular food as if it were toxic. The body's tissues then produce chemicals such as histamine to deal with the 'toxin'.

Approximately 90 per cent of food allergies are produced by cow's milk, hen's eggs, nuts, soy, wheat, fish and shellfish, while the remaining 10 per cent are caused by other foods. Food allergies are much more common in children than adults, and more often than not will diminish with age. The symptoms of food allergies include headaches, breathing problems, stomach upsets and skin rashes, and some of these can potentially be life-threatening.

FOOD INTOLERANCES

Unlike food allergies, food intolerances are not caused by the immune system reacting to a food, but are in essence a chemical reaction to a substance in a particular food that causes various symptoms. Whether a food intolerance is going to be a temporary or lifelong problem will depend on the particular food and the reason your child's body is reacting to it. The most common food intolerances are caused by dairy, strawberries, citrus fruits, tomatoes, food additives and foods containing histamines.

Compared to allergies, intolerance reactions are generally less severe, but they can still cause a lot of discomfort. In some cases, if only a small amount of the food has been consumed, symptoms may go unnoticed. Over time, repeated exposure to foods causing intolerance can lead to conditions including asthma, chronic fatigue syndrome and irritable bowel syndrome.

DIAGNOSING FOOD ALLERGIES AND INTOLERANCES

If you think your child might have an allergy or intolerance to a particular food, ask for a professional diagnosis from your GP or integrative specialist, who can refer you to an allergy clinic. Commercial allergy-testing kits can be unreliable, so it's best to have the results interpreted by a health professional. The Australian Society of Clinical Immunology and Allergy (allergy.org.au), Allergy UK (allergyuk.org) and the Asthma and Allergy Foundation of America (aafa.org) all have useful information on food allergies and intolerances.

This book has specific recipes suitable for certain allergies – check the symbols (see pages 42–44) above each recipe.

HIDDEN SUGARS

When looking at ingredients lists, remember that sugar could be disguised as any of the following:

agave
brown sugar
cane sugar
confectioners' sugar
corn syrup
demerara sugar
fructose
galactose
granulated sugar
grape sugar
high-fructose
  corn syrup

high-maltose
  corn syrup
honey
invert sugar
lactose
malt
maltodextrin
maltose
maple syrup
molasses
muscovado sugar
palm sugar

panela
refined sugar
rice syrup
sucrose
table sugar
treacle
turbinado sugar
white sugar

TIPS FOR REMOVING SUGAR AND ADDITIVES

Sugar consumption in our society has dramatically contributed to the deteriorating health of our population. Dr Robert Lustig, a world expert on childhood obesity and Professor of Pediatrics in the Division of Endocrinology at the University of California, urges us to re-evaluate our role as consumers of sugar and identify how hidden sugars find their way into our diet. He suggests that not all calories are created equal, as different foods are metabolised in different ways, and that calories from sugars such as fructose can have significant harmful consequences for children's health and wellbeing.

Highly addictive for children, sugar is carefully hidden in everyday food and products by manufacturers (see the box opposite). We have all seen how it can transform even the quietest and most measured child into a screaming nightmare. Biologically, sugar can suppress the immune system; contribute to hyperactivity, anxiety, depression, and concentration and learning difficulties; promote tooth decay, food allergies and their symptoms; and influence a host of other conditions.

Although recent studies have established a correlation between sugar-rich foods and childhood behavioural problems, many parents still struggle to get their kids' sugar addictions under control.

It's not always possible to eliminate sugar completely, but replacing it with healthy alternatives is the next best step. If your child is stuck on sugar and processed foods, try these tips.

STEP 1: START IN YOUR OWN BACKYARD

Think about how your own food choices affect your children, and look at what you and your partner or your family are eating. Are you nutrition role models for your children? Or have you filled your pantry and fridge with health-sabotaging foods such as cake mixes, deep-fried foods and chips; sugar-laden cereals, biscuits, cakes, pastries and crackers; and foods containing bad fats such as vegetable oil, hydrogenated oils and margarine?

STEP 2: CLEAN OUT THE CUPBOARDS

Packaged and processed foods can look tempting in the shop, but try not to rely on them as pantry fillers. Many are full of sugars, bad fats, additives and preservatives that have a negative effect on children. Go through your pantry and throw out the worst offenders first. If you have some moderately offending foods just let them run out naturally and slowly introduce new, healthier versions.

STEP 3: KNOW WHAT THEY'RE EATING

Check labels for hidden sugars cleverly disguised under assorted names (see page 16) depending on the processing methods used to produce them. Also look for foods containing artificial ingredients, chemicals and additives (see pages 22–23). If a food has a long list of ingredients, avoid it. The magic number for ingredients on a label is five or less – in other words, make sure you can count the ingredients on one hand.

Scrutinise labels and check the fine print for hidden ingredients. Unfortunately, not all ingredients are always declared on labels. Our food-labelling laws allow manufacturers to leave an ingredient off the list if the amount falls below a certain percentage, but just do the best you can. If your child is on an extremely strict elimination diet, you can contact the manufacturer to obtain a full ingredients list.

STEP 4: INTRODUCE HEALTHIER CHOICES

Once you've eliminated the controversial foods from your cupboards, start introducing healthier options. Breakfast is generally the hardest meal to replace if your kids are used to eating sweetened cereals. If this is the case, have on hand natural, sugar-free options, such as puffed rice, buckwheat and quinoa cereals. Try adding sliced banana or berries or rice malt syrup to sweeten them as you're introducing new foods. Just take it slowly with small swaps and don't try to make too many sudden changes or you might have a mutiny on your hands! Oats make delicious porridge. Pancake mixes can be made up ahead of time, and sliced bread can be frozen ready to toast on busy mornings. Eggs and soldiers make a fun breakfast, as do homemade baked beans on toast.

For pantry staples, look for soups, stocks, low-salt tinned beans, tuna and salmon, coconut milk and tomato purées with no additives or sugar. Keep a supply of rice crackers and gluten-free grains and seeds such as brown rice, quinoa and buckwheat. Research shows that children are more likely to eat what they help pick out at the supermarket, so take them along and make them part of the process. Encourage them to try some new colours and textures, and make up fun names for vegetables and dishes such as X-ray vision carrots or Rockin' fried rice (page 119).

GOOD FATS AND BAD FATS

Natural fats and oils are vital for healthy immune function. The best oils to use are coconut oil, cold-pressed extra virgin olive oil, fish oils and organic butter.

Good fats increase the body's ability to absorb nutrients from foods and also provide your body with energy. They're fantastic at helping the body eliminate heavy metals such as aluminium, mercury, nickel and lead. Eating good fats can cleanse the entire body as well as rebuild cell membranes. Good fats also act as carriers for the important fat-soluble vitamins A, D, E and K, and aid in the conversion of carotene to vitamin A.

The most damaging fats and oils for the body are man-made hydrogenated fats (trans fats) and polyunsaturated fats from vegetable oils. These fats and oils affect the structure of our cells and severely depress the immune system.

Avoid oils derived from plants, such as canola (rapeseed), soybean, safflower, sunflower and corn. Many processed foods contain these fats and oils, such as margarine, salad dressing, mayonnaise, cakes and biscuits. These fats are not always listed on the ingredients label. If unsure, stop eating processed foods and whenever possible eat wholesome, fresh ingredients.

 SUPERCHARGED TIP Food that's off limits is tempting for kids. If you want to give your child potato chips, choose a brand with good-quality natural ingredients.

ALTERNATIVE SWEETENERS

You can give white processed sugar the boot by introducing alternative sugars and sweeteners. Just a word of warning: these substitutes can spark sugar cravings. You'll read conflicting reports about which sugar alternative is best, so find one that works for your family and use it in the recipes. Don't forget you can also use real fruit in recipes to sweeten them.

 SUPERCHARGED TIP To break it down, a quick way of remembering what constitutes a sugar on an ingredients list is that anything ending in -ose is a sugar, while anything ending in -ol is a sugar alcohol, and dextrins, syrups and juice concentrates are also forms of sugars.

✱ **STEVIA** My sweetener of choice is stevia, which is a perennial plant native to Paraguay and Brazil. The sweetness comes from the leaves, which are crushed or distilled to create a powder or syrup. Stevia is a lot sweeter than traditional sugars, so you only need to use a fraction of the amount. It can be purchased at health food stores and online, and is now readily available in larger supermarkets. When using stevia, the golden rule is 1 cup of sugar is equivalent to 1 teaspoon of stevia liquid and powder, and 1 tablespoon is equivalent to ¼ teaspoon or about 8 drops. A teaspoon of sugar equates to a pinch of powder or 3 drops of liquid. Look for one without a bitter aftertaste – it's so important to find one that you can work with and that kids will enjoy.

✱ **XYLITOL** This sugar substitute found naturally in fibrous fruits and vegies such as plums and corn is also produced naturally in the body. Xylitol is metabolised slowly, so it won't cause the 'sugar spikes' (suddenly elevated blood sugar) that can be experienced with other sugar products. For some children it can cause stomach pain and can have a laxative effect when taken in excess, so it needs to be tested in small quantities first. One reason it's a good alternative to sugar is that it promotes oral health and prevents tooth decay. In a 2004 study, researchers also found that xylitol damages *Streptococcus* *pneumoniae*, one of the main causes of ear infections, by preventing the bacteria from multiplying. It's a handy ingredient to use in baking, and the volume ratio to sugar is one to one, but start by adding half the amount and do a taste test when making the recipes.

✴ **RICE MALT SYRUP** This syrup has the sweetness of caramelised honey. When using rice malt syrup in recipes, use the same volume as you would of sugar. Rice malt syrup is made by culturing rice with enzymes to break down the starches and then the mixture is cooked until it becomes a syrup. Unlike fructose, it provides a steady supply of energy to the body from a mixture of complex carbohydrates, maltose and a small amount of glucose.

✴ **COCONUT SUGAR** This low-GI sugar doesn't cause sugar spikes and, although it contains fructose, it also has other health benefits. It is derived from the sap of the coconut palm flower, and contains minerals and amino acids such as glutamic acid, which is an important component in metabolism and acts as a neurotransmitter.

✴ **DEXTROSE (GLUCOSE)** This simple monosaccharide (single sugar) is made by plants and our cells use it as their primary source of energy. You can purchase it as a powder and use it in baking. A word of caution: because dextrose is glucose, it has a very high glycemic index, entering our system directly through the gut wall and into the bloodstream. It raises blood sugar levels and stimulates a high insulin response very quickly.

✴ **HONEY** Honey makes a great alternative to sugar.

*Positive reinforcement is a great tool –
remember to praise children when
they try a new food*

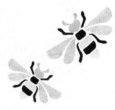

AVOIDING ADDITIVES

The table opposite lists some of the common additives that cause problems and are best avoided. Note that the numbers will also sometimes appear with an 'E' in front of them.

Adverse reactions to additives in children can vary, but some of the signs to look for are:

✳ **DIGESTIVE** diarrhoea, abdominal pain, colicky pains
✳ **NERVOUS SYSTEM** hyperactivity, insomnia, irritability
✳ **RESPIRATORY** asthma, sinusitis, rhinitis
✳ **SKIN** itching, hives, rashes and swelling.

If you think your child may have a food-additive sensitivity, trying to avoid the additive and keeping a food diary will help. Note down any adverse reactions and eliminate the suspected allergen. It's best to consult your medical practitioner if reactions continue, as it could be a sign of other disorders.

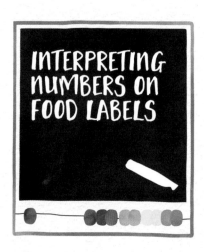

INTERPRETING NUMBERS ON FOOD LABELS

COMMON ADDITIVES ON FOOD LABELS

ARTIFICIAL COLOURS
102 Tartrazine
107 Yellow 2G
110 Sunset yellow
120 Carmines, Cochineal
122 Azorubine, Carmoisine
123 Amaranth (red)
124 Ponceau, Brilliant scarlet
127 Erythrosine (red)
129 Allura red AC
132 Indigotine, Indigo carmine
133 Brilliant blue
142 Green S
143 Fast green
150 Caramel
151 Brilliant black
155 Brown
160b Annatto

PRESERVATIVES
173 Aluminium
200–203 Sorbates
210–217 Benzoates
220–228 Sulfites
249–252 Nitrates, Nitrites
260 Acetic acid
280–283 Propionates

ANTIOXIDANTS
310–312 Gallates
319 Tert-butylhydroquinone
   (TBHQ)
320 Butylated hydroxyanisole
   (BHA)
321 Butylated hydroxytoluene
   (BHT)

THICKENERS, STABILISERS, EMULSIFIERS, SWEETENERS, ANTICAKING AGENTS
407 Carrageenan
413 Tragacanth gum
414 Acacia gum, Gum arabic
416 Karaya gum
421 Mannitol
431 Polyoxylethylene (40) stearate
433, 435–436 Polysorbates
441 Gelatine
466 Sodium carboxymethylcellulose
507 Hydrochloric acid
518 Magnesium sulfate
536 Potassium ferrocyanide
553 Talc
903 Carnauba wax (used in chewing gums)
905 Paraffin, Vaseline, White mineral oil
924 Potassium bromate (used in bleaching flour)
925 Chlorine (used in bleaching flour)
926 Chlorine dioxide (used in bleaching flour and
   as a preservative)
928 Benzoyl peroxide (used in bleaching flour and
   as a bread enhancer)
950 Acesulfame potassium (sweetener)
951 Aspartame (sweetener)
952 Cyclamate, Cyclamic acid (sweeteners)
954 Saccharine (sweetener)
1202 Polyvinylpyrrolidone (added to pharmaceuticals)
1403 Bleached starch

FLAVOUR ENHANCERS
620–625 Glutamates such
   as MSG
627 Disodium guanylate
631 Disodium inosinate
635 Disodium ribonucleotides

OTHERS TO AVOID
Hydrolysed vegetable protein
   (HVP)
All artificial flavours
Whey powder in bread

PACKING AND PRESENTING A CREATIVE LUNCHBOX

When it comes to packing school lunches your kids will enjoy and devour, much of the battle will be in communication and variety. Unfortunately, taking the 'You'll get what you're given' approach that many of us may have experienced is a surefire way to ensure that kids are removed from a positive, *relational* experience of food.

What we're all aiming for is a place where children are able to engage freely and creatively in the process of making healthy food choices, and to learn how to take responsibility for what they're eating. Opening up a two-way conversation about the importance of eating real foods, and giving your kids the opportunity to make some choices about what they might have in their lunchbox, will more likely result in an empty container on their return home from school.

Let your child be involved in the purchase of their lunchbox. Make sure it's sturdy, with a strong lid, and is insulated or comes with an icepack – no parent likes a black mushy banana on the return trip home. Choose a lunchbox with separate compartments and make sure it's large enough to hold a flask or drink bottle. Using smaller airtight containers will protect the lunchbox and its contents, and alleviate the need for foil and plastic wrap. They're useful for dips, salads, fruit, wraps and casseroles.

When attempting to expose your kids to new, more nutrient-dense real foods, it's a no-brainer that a dull, monochromatic spread of food is unlikely to entice their tastebuds. We eat not only with our

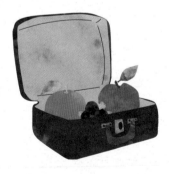

mouths, but first and foremost with our *eyes*, so presenting a visually appealing, colourful lunchbox is a must.

A nutritionally balanced lunchbox should contain an array of food from various food groups. Use different types of fruit and vegetables; seeds; coconut flakes; full-fat calcium-rich dairy foods; and protein-rich foods such as meats, eggs, nut butters, pulses and oily fish such as tuna. You'll find a bunch of healthy bread options here, including wraps and pittas, which are a good source of long-term energy.

 SUPERCHARGED TIP Make a 'rainbow salad' with different-coloured ingredients, such as purple cabbage, red tomatoes, green snow peas (mangetout), orange carrot and yellow capsicum (pepper).

SIMPLE STRATEGIES FOR A HEALTHY LUNCHBOX

A few simple substitutions will improve your child's diet enormously. If in doubt, remember to try to choose natural, whole and real foods.

Use real butter instead of margarine; full-fat dairy in place of low-fat, which is often packed with sugar and additives; real cheese instead of plastic cheese slices; and organic meats where possible. Major supermarkets now carry very affordable organic meat. When it comes to legumes, buy dried beans, which are more economical than canned.

Using real food will teach your child to appreciate food's natural flavours and develop an understanding of what real food actually tastes like. Try to skip the sugar-filled, artificially flavoured yoghurts in the supermarket and instead opt for full-cream plain yoghurt with mixed fresh berries in a fun container with an animal-shaped spoon. You can turn it into chocolate yoghurt by adding raw cacao powder and a touch of natural sweetener, or try a mini avocado and chocolate mousse. Adding flavourless chia seeds to yoghurt will provide sustenance as well as essential protein, calcium, vitamin C, iron, potassium and omega-3 essential fatty acids. You can add seeds to trail mixes too, along with coconut flakes, vitamin C–rich goji berries and dehydrated fruit.

Making kids' lunches interactive and less soggy is also important. Separate dry and wet ingredients such as homemade dressings, sauces, spreads and slices of tomato for crackers and sandwiches in mini containers, and let the kids engage in some of the preparation of the food. Mix up textures of smooth yoghurt with crunchy pepitas (pumpkin seeds), or gluten-free sandwiches with contrasting fillings of creamy avocado, slinky sprouts, crunchy slivers of celery and a homemade mayo. Homemade soups can be frozen in single portions and then reheated in the morning and placed in a thermos for lunchbox use. Incorporate dinner leftovers into lunch the next day. Grains, meats, vegetables, eggs and undressed salads all make excellent additions to a lunchbox.

When it comes to drinks, rather than providing a reconstituted fruit juice, why not try a 'green monster', blending green vegies such as kale, spinach and cucumber with apple, pear and lemon juice for an exciting, eye-catching beverage. Flasks of chocolate milk can be made at home with rice or almond milk and raw cacao powder. Banana smoothies help kids feel full for longer.

Always encourage your child to drink water – it hydrates, regulates body temperature, and helps prevent constipation and urinary tract infections. It's also important for your child's oral health, immune system, digestion and weight management. To make it fun for them, give them a straw, and add some ice and a squeeze of fresh lemon or a mint leaf to give it a hint of flavour. You could even drop in a couple of frozen berries. If you're still having trouble getting your child to drink more water, set them a pee challenge – the lighter the pee the better.

For healthy lunchboxes it's always a good idea to keep a variety of fresh fruit and vegies in stock. Having raw fruit and veg that you can simply cut up is the easiest way to ensure your kids are snacking on fresh, nutrient-rich foods. Eating seasonal fruit and vegetables that are in abundance will be less of a strain on the purse strings.

 SUPERCHARGED TIP Keep pre-cut celery, cucumber, carrot and capsicum (pepper) in the fridge for incredibly quick last-minute snacks or as a colourful addition to school lunchboxes.

TIPS FOR BUSY FAMILIES

It's great to be organised with meal planning and cooking so you can spend more quality time with the kids. Schedule an hour a week to organise your meals and shopping list (see pages 45–47) for the week ahead – putting in some clever prep will save you time and money in the long run. Include your kids in the planning so they can develop an appreciation of and look forward to the meals to come.

Choose meals for the whole week that will satisfy the health needs and preferences of all the family, and write a matching shopping list. If you want to be really organised, map out three weeks' worth of meal plans and shopping lists, and rotate them.

It's a good idea to cook meals the whole family can enjoy. Why prepare a completely separate meal for your kids if they can get in on Mum and Dad's? Roast dinners, soups and casseroles can be enjoyed by kids and adults alike.

Remember to make the most of a single ingredient. Getting to know how you can use a single food item for multiple meal ideas will save you large amounts of time and money. If you ever come across a cheap, high-quality staple ingredient that can be used in a variety of family meals, buy up and brainstorm recipe ideas for future meals and kids' lunchbox options.

A TIME-SAVING BAKING MIX

Find a 'universal baking mix' and keep it on hand. A basic baking mix that takes into consideration any allergies or sensitivities will be a lifesaver for a busy parent. Keep a dry mixture in a big container, and experiment with whatever seasonal or available additions you have in the kitchen. Sneak in vegies such as roasted pumpkin with spinach and seeds for a savoury option, or frozen blueberries with shredded coconut and stevia for a healthy sweet fix. Get creative – the possibilities are endless!

This fantastic gluten-free self-raising baking mix is a great all-rounder to keep in the pantry. Combine these ingredients and store in an airtight container.

150 g (5½ oz/1½ cups) blanched almond meal
95 g (3¼ oz/¾ cup) tapioca flour (arrowroot)
25 g (1 oz/¼ cup) flaxseed meal
½ teaspoon Celtic sea salt
1 teaspoon baking powder
¼ teaspoon bicarbonate of soda (baking soda)

 SUPERCHARGED TIP For an even simpler mix, combine 125 g (4½ oz/¾ cup) rice flour, 25 g (1 oz/¼ cup) almond meal and 1½ teaspoons gluten-free baking powder.

BATCH COOKING AND LEFTOVERS

Fancy an escape to the kitchen for a few hours? Have you ever tried make-ahead batch cooking? All you need to do is prioritise one day every couple of weeks for a batch-cooking session based around whatever seasonal produce or ingredients you have on hand. Preparing freezable items such as soups, stews, curries, homemade pizza bases, stocks, dips, breads, muffins and slices will save huge amounts of time when preparing lunchboxes and midweek meals. Include prep for your week's meals on these days as well: chop and bag vegies, and make staples such as sauces and spice mixes that you'll need during the busy days ahead.

 SUPERCHARGED TIP Knock up batches of from-scratch soups, casseroles, bolognese and stews to fill your freezer with homemade midweek meals.

It's a good idea to make popsicles and mini frozen treats (see page 143) as a healthier alternative to ice cream. Kids absolutely *love* icy treats. Fill iceblock (popsicle/ice lolly) or push-up moulds with blended fruit or mixtures of homemade fruit and vegetable juices for a nutrient-rich sweet treat. Freeze concoctions in smaller portions in your everyday ice-cube tray, and present them to your kids as 'ice lollies'. They won't even notice the difference between your homemade goods and the chemical-laden iceblocks from the corner shop.

 SUPERCHARGED TIP Blend a banana and freeze it as a wholesome, delicious ice cream mimic! Or try freezing natural yoghurt with whole berries.

If you have a busy day ahead, use last night's dinner leftovers for the next day's breakfast and lunch. It's amazing how many home-cooked dinner leftovers can be creatively added to omelettes, salads or toasted sandwiches, or made into interesting mini pizza toppings for kids' breakfast and lunch options the next day. Present last night's bolognese between slices of scrumptious sourdough or gluten-free bread, or leftover stewed fruits on top of a morning muesli.

To ensure you spend time together, combine family time with food-preparation time. Allow your kids to unleash their creative side in the kitchen while you're prepping meals. Involving children and teaching them the art of home cooking provides them with the opportunity to appreciate the meals they have at home. Give kids the option of adorning their own mini pizzas, or of adding different 'sprinkles' to their morning muesli, such as chia, hemp and flaxseeds, goji berries and other nutrient-rich toppings.

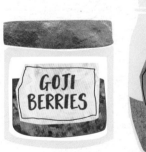
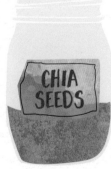

SNEAKING EVERYDAY SUPERFOODS INTO KIDS' MEALS

I'm always suspicious of parents who say their kids eat everything. Is it really true? And what's their secret? Most kids go through phases – they eat whatever you put in front of them at first, then they develop a taste for things and start rejecting anything that isn't pasta (or so it seems). The green vegies are often the first to go, while the orange ones linger a little longer, and eggplant (aubergine) or mushrooms never get much of a look-in! Here are six ways to sneak superfoods into your child's diet.

✱ **SECRET SPINACH SMOOTHIE** Next time you make a blueberry smoothie (an excellent source of antioxidants), toss in a handful of spinach and it will likely go undetected.

 SUPERCHARGED TIP Blend a handful of spinach with a scoop of Greek-style yoghurt, a scoop of ice, blueberries, half a banana and almond or rice milk.

✱ **MARINARA SAUCE** Most kids love pasta, so take advantage of it and make a sauce that's full of vegetables. When cooking the sauce as you normally would, add zucchini (courgette), broccoli, cauliflower, kale or any other vegetable you'd like to sneak in. Blend the sauce smooth before dishing it up with a bowl of pasta.

✱ **VEGIE-PACKED MEATBALLS** Next time you make meatballs, use a food processor to blend mushrooms and zucchini, then add it to the meat mixture before forming the balls. Once the meatballs are cooked, your kids won't notice the extra vegies, but you'll know they're there! Try the recipe for Vegie-packed lamb meatballs on page 104.

✱ **CAULIFLOWER MASH** This white vegie is not an easy one to get kids to eat whole. Mashed, however, it's a whole new ball game. Mashed cauliflower is one of the most delicious side dishes a parent can make. Add a potato or two (if you like) to maintain texture, and your kids will love it.

 SUPERCHARGED TIP Sneak puréed cauliflower into a white creamy sauce and pour it over grilled chicken breast.

✱ **CHIA MUFFINS** Chia seeds are a delicious superfood, packed with omega-3s and ridiculously high in antioxidants. They're extremely versatile and easy to use. Add them to smoothies, sprinkle on top of yoghurt or muesli, or toss them into your muffin mix. When mixed with water, chia seeds become gelatinous. In this form you can use them as an egg substitute in your baking recipes.

✱ **DIP IT** Kids love an interactive meal! Making their own anything always goes down well. They seem especially to enjoy dips. Surround a nice healthy dip (see pages 98–101) with carrot sticks, celery sticks, snow peas (mangetout) and cucumber slices, and you're bound to increase their vegie quotient quickly.

HUMMUS AND GUACAMOLE
are perfect for dipping carrot and celery sticks

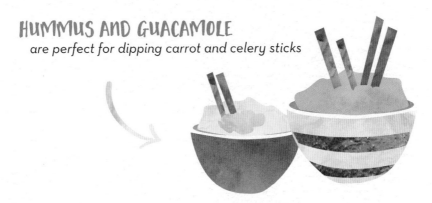

MOOD FOOD:
AVOIDING THE CRAZIES

Our children's little bodies are sensitive to what they eat, and food can quickly affect their mood. We've all seen it happen – a dozen children going crazy at a party. They get doped up on fairy bread and strung out on lollies. Then there's the post-party meltdown, when tears flow and moodiness creeps in. If your child's diet is full of junk food, they won't receive the nutrients their brain needs for healthy neurotransmitter function. On top of that, our brains need fuel to transmit the messages that control our feelings and emotions.

Some children are more susceptible to mood alterations from an unhealthy diet. The mood swings they experience can ultimately affect their behaviour, learning abilities, and relationships with their peers and family.

Foods with low nutrient profiles and allergenic ingredients can cause behavioural changes in some sensitive children. Children with attention deficit hyperactivity disorder (ADHD) have existing behavioural problems that can be aggravated by certain foods.

Stabilise your child's mood by offering them a well-balanced and varied diet filled with real and nutrient-dense foods. The first thing you need to do to control your child's mood is remove foods with additives and added sugar (see pages 17–23). Next, increase their intake of fruit and vegetables, then boost their levels of essential fats. Try introducing the following good-mood foods.

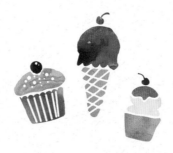

✸ B-VITAMIN FOODS Studies show that low levels of B vitamins may be linked to depression, so maintaining a steady level of intake could help keep our mood stable. One of the best sources of vitamin B is eggs. Other great sources include fish, chicken and meat.

 SUPERCHARGED TIP Unless your child is allergic, eggs are a quick and easy go-to dinner. Serve them boiled or scrambled, with brown toast spread with avocado.

✸ DOPAMINE-HEAVY FOODS Dopamine is a natural feel-good chemical in the brain that plays a role in the pleasure and reward pathways. Foods that can boost dopamine levels include almonds, avocados, bananas, pepitas (pumpkin seeds) and dairy products.

 SUPERCHARGED TIP Create a picture on your child's plate using a cut-up banana, sliced avocado, almonds and pepitas. Serve it with a glass of almond or rice milk for the perfect dopamine-heavy snack.

✸ FOLIC ACID FOODS Folic acid is a B vitamin (see above) yet it's such an essential mood-booster, it deserves a special shout-out. Foods high in folic acid are the dark, leafy vegies that many kids won't go near. These include spinach, kale, asparagus, broccoli and brussels sprouts.

 SUPERCHARGED TIP Blend, blend, blend. Puréeing dark leafy greens is a great way to sneak them into a tomato-based pasta sauce, or shred them and sneak them into a spinach bread or savoury muffins.

✸ FISH OILS Your child's brain and nervous system need a good supply of fat to function and develop effectively. A number of fats – such as the trans fats found in processed meats and deep-fried foods – are detrimental to health, but others are essential, and a deficiency could negatively impact a child's behaviour. One study found that the omega-3 fatty acids in fish oil increase the levels in the brain of serotonin, a neurotransmitter that controls emotion. This makes fish oils a very good mood food to include in your child's diet. Along with tuna and salmon, try to include spinach and sunflower seeds in your recipes, as these also contain omega-3 fatty acids. Tuna can be snuck into a marinara sauce, salmon can be used in salmon bake, and spinach and seeds can be thrown into smoothies. A tablespoon of seeds tossed on muesli or sprinkled on soups or salads every day will provide your child with essential good fats.

 SUPERCHARGED TIP Seed mixes can be ground in a coffee grinder and kept in a glass jar in the fridge.

✦ **COMPLEX CARBOHYDRATES** Not all carbohydrates are created equal. Avoid the sugary, white-bread processed carbs that often dominate the party spread (think doughnuts, soft drink, fairy bread), and instead opt for sourdough bread, brown rice and fruit. These complex-carb foods are less likely to create the crazy ups and downs than processed foods because they don't wreak such havoc on blood sugar levels.

 SUPERCHARGED TIP A hummus dip with brown rice bread fingers is a great snack for kids. Pair it with a fruit platter and you can call it lunch.

Foods with low nutrient profiles and allergenic ingredients can cause behavioural changes in some sensitive children.

CONCENTRATION, LET'S BEGIN!

For kids, the school day is long and they work nonstop. From running around the playground to learning maths, reading, art and sport – our kids are busy! You can help them stay focused and alert by feeding them good foods. Here are some ideas.

✴ **CEREALS** Oats are a great, long-lasting energy source that will help your child stay all ears until recess. Choose an unflavoured oatmeal or untoasted muesli (to cut down on sugar) and sprinkle sulfur-free dried fruit, nuts, chia seeds or flaxseeds on top. A dollop of natural sugar-free, full-fat yoghurt will create a creamy texture, while some grated apple will add sweetness and boost the fibre content. In winter, a quinoa porridge with berries goes down a treat; you'll find one on page 63.

✴ **EGGS** These always get a mention when we're talking healthy, energy-sustaining foods, and they come up trumps for concentration, too. The fat and protein settle the brain and allow for attentiveness. It's the perfect combination. Try my Cheesy mini tartlets (page 56) or Cheesy bacon and egg scramble (page 62).

✴ **FRUIT AND NUTS** When a slump hits, a lovely juicy orange can provide the natural glucose a child's brain needs to get back on track. Accompany it with a handful of almonds or walnuts to create the ideal brain-boosting snack. Many schools have a nut-free policy due to allergies, so keep them as breakfast food before school or as an after-school snack. Walnuts contain omega-3s and almonds are high in B vitamins and magnesium, which all boost brain function. The Breakfast yoghurt fruit cocktail on page 62 is a great way for kids to start the day.

✶ **AVOCADO** Just like the egg, the avocado is one of nature's perfect foods. Full of good-for-you fats and long-lasting protein, avocado is a must-have food when you're talking about brain function. Try spreading it on toast in place of butter, or try an avocado and banana wrap – a smooth concoction that will definitely fill the hunger void. It even tastes good on yummy Banana bread (page 128). Kids can also dip away on Guacamole (page 101).

✶ **BLUEBERRIES** If you're not already eating blueberries every day, you should be! Not only are they delicious, but they pack a punch when it comes to brain-enhancing antioxidants. Use frozen blueberries instead of fresh if they're out of season: toss a handful on your breakfast cereal or make a blueberry smoothie as an afternoon snack (try the Very berry shake on page 52).

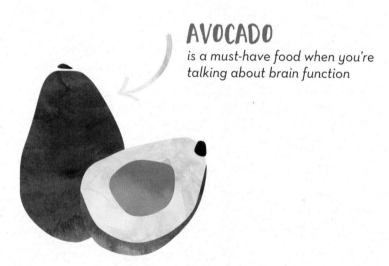

AVOCADO
is a must-have food when you're talking about brain function

ENERGY AND PERFORMANCE FOOD

Kids can be like the Energizer Bunny – they keep going and going and going and then just conk out. Giving them foods that will help burn optimal energy so they can finish the race on a high is the ideal way to help them perform at their best. The trick is to provide them with sustainable energy throughout the day rather than energy that will burn out and leave them exhausted and depleted. It's time to say goodbye to energy and sports drinks – which are full of sugar, artificial ingredients and chemicals – and say hello to some of these healthy food ideas.

✱ **CHICKEN DRUMMERS** Next time you're at the supermarket, pick up a few packs of organic chicken drumsticks. Bake them at home and keep them in the fridge for a quick energy-boosting snack. As long as you're sure your child's lunchbox will be kept cool, you can pop them in their school lunch, too. The Crunchy chicken drummers on page 105 are simple to make.

 SUPERCHARGED TIP Try coating chicken with a crunchy coconut or seed mix.

✱ **AVOCADO SPREAD** Most kids don't mind avocado – it's fairly bland and won't shock their tastebuds. Spread some between some gluten-free crackers for a protein-rich snack that fills them up. Add a layer of almond butter for an extra protein boost.

✱ **SALMON** Salmon is so jam-packed with omega-3 fats and protein that it's worth getting your kids used to eating it. If your kids don't scream 'Yum!' when they hear fish is on the menu, all is not lost. Try my Mini salmon frittatas (page 109) for starters.

 SUPERCHARGED TIP Buy salmon fillets and use a food processor to mince them, then add coconut, egg, lemon juice and fresh parsley. Form into cakes and cook in a lightly oiled frying pan. Serve with steamed broccoli for a delicious and healthy dinner.

✱ **SKEWER IT UP!** With kids, it's all about presentation. Grab a few skewers and thread on alternating cubes of cheese and bite-sized pieces of fruit. You can even add chunks of cooked chicken for a skewer that's not only fun to eat but provides all the protein your child needs to get through the afternoon.

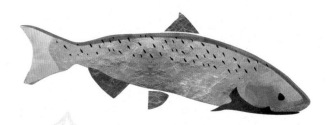

SALMON
is so jam-packed with omega-3 fats and protein that it's worth getting your kids used to eating it

SQUAD FOOD

If you pick your kids up from school and then go on to Little Athletics, basketball, soccer, netball or any other sport or activity – music lessons, say – for a few hours before home time, you'll need some nutritious snacks to get them through the afternoon. Not only are kids always starving after school, but they need something yummy that will give them energy to perform at their best.

Having nutritious, energy-filled snacks on hand requires a bit of planning, but it needn't be too time-consuming. Here are a few tips.

✹ **HEALTHY SMOOTHIE** This makes the perfect afternoon pick-up snack and will fill the void between lunch and dinner while your child does whatever afternoon activity takes their fancy. Blend sugar-free vanilla yoghurt with seeds and a handful of fresh berries.

✹ **FRIED RICE** If you're making a stir-fry for dinner during the week, always cook up ample brown rice for leftovers. Combine the rice in a pan with anything you've got in the fridge – peas, diced leftover chicken, grated carrot and scrambled egg. Toss in a bit of wheat-free tamari for a tasty, protein-filled afternoon snack. Rockin' fried rice (page 119) is a good option.

✹ **TUNA WRAP** Tuna doesn't always last well in a school lunchbox, but make it just before you pick up the kids from school and it'll stay fresh in the car in a cooled lunchbox. Spread avocado over a wrap and spoon tuna on top. Add a few crunchy lettuce leaves, wrap it up and there's a wholesome snack that's good to go.

✹ **EGGS** Hard-boiled eggs are the perfect snack before sports training. Pre-peel them so they're quick to eat. Add a handful of nuts and an apple to make an unbeatable protein-filled snack.

✹ **SUSHI** Brown rice sushi is a great after-school snack. Filled with cooked tuna, salmon, avocado or cucumber, sushi will satisfy that empty tummy and provide long-lasting energy to burn.

PART TWO
RECIPES

A GUIDE TO THE ICONS

▲ WF WHEAT-FREE

Wheat is found in products such as breads and cereals, prepared mixtures such as pancakes and waffles, biscuits and crackers, cereal beverages, salad dressings, sauces such as soy, luncheon meats, malted milk, modified starches, tinned soups and crumbed vegetable products. For some children, wheat is hard to digest and can cause allergic reactions such as urticaria (hives) and anaphylaxis. Other common symptoms of a wheat allergy include eczema, asthma, hay fever, irritable bowel syndrome, bloated stomach, tummy aches, nausea, headaches, joint pain, depression, mood swings and tiredness. Wheat products can be replaced with buckwheat, rice, quinoa, tapioca and wheat-free flours.

▲ DF DAIRY-FREE

In Australia, New Zealand, the United Kingdom and the United States, 2-5 per cent of babies are allergic to cow's milk and dairy products. Dairy allergy can be confirmed by your doctor using allergy tests, such as skin-prick tests or blood tests. To avoid dairy in the supermarket, look on labels for any food that contains cow's or goat's milk, cheese, butter, ghee, buttermilk, cream, crème fraîche, milk powder, whey, casein, caseinate and margarines that contain milk products. Allergic symptoms in children may include hives, eczema, face swelling, vomiting, diarrhoea, and noisy breathing or wheezing. Substitutes for dairy milk can include rice milk, nut milks, oat milk and coconut milk.

▲ GF GLUTEN-FREE

Gluten is a mixture of proteins found in grains such as wheat, rye, barley and oats. Some children can tolerate oats, but the tricky bit is finding oats that haven't been contaminated with wheat or other grains during processing. Symptoms of gluten sensitivity in children can include growing pains, chronic ear infections, eczema, agitation and mood swings, changes in weight, dental problems, headaches, depression, and gastrointestinal issues. Gluten sensitivity can make your child feel ill or uncomfortable a lot of the time, and can affect their mood and quality of life. Gluten-sensitive children may experience slow growth due to their inability to absorb essential nutrients.

▲ SF SUGAR-FREE

Sugar is addictive and it's everywhere, from muesli bars to yoghurt and even tinned peas, sausages and tomato sauce. Some of the worst offenders are the between-meal snacks or drinks; these affect a child's appetite and can contribute to stunted growth, and behavioural and dental problems. Sugar can also contribute to nutrient deficiencies, as it provides energy without any of the nutrients required by growing bodies. Researchers have shown that a child with vitamin and mineral deficiencies such as magnesium, zinc, fatty acids and B-group vitamins are more than likely to show symptoms of ADHD and behavioural problems. Some children have trouble digesting certain sugars. This affects their internal gut flora, causing loose bowel actions and/or constipation, and making them more prone to a build-up of bad bacteria in the gut and yeast (candida) infections. Try putting nutrient-dense snacks first if you're looking for a quick fix to silence cries for sugar-filled treats in the most awkward places. Remember that both a can of cola and a bottle of apple juice contain about 10 teaspoons of sugar each.

▲ VG VEGETARIAN

These recipes are suitable for vegans and contain no animal products. To ensure your child is eating enough of the essential nutrients needed for growth, make sure you include other forms of protein, iron, vitamin B12, vitamin D and calcium in their diet. Good fats from non-meat sources are also very important. It's essential for parents to encourage children to eat a wide variety of foods and not cut out whole food groups unless absolutely necessary.

▲ NF NUT-FREE

This symbol indicates that the recipe does not contain nuts in any form although it may contain seeds. If it's accompanied by an asterisk, the recipe can be modified to be nut-free. Substitutes for nuts can include sesame, poppy and sunflower seeds and pepitas (pumpkin seeds). Nuts can be found in cereals, sauces, health bars, crackers and biscuits, baked goods, pesto, chocolates and ice cream. The lunchbox meals are all nut-free to satisfy the no-nut policy of many schools.

THE SILVER LINING? You get to experiment in the kitchen with new ingredients and find fun ways to nourish your child with real food.

MAKING A SHOPPING LIST

Forward planning and organisation make feeding children much easier. Keep a list up on the fridge of what you need to buy for the week. You could also try one of the free smartphone shopping list apps.

Use the list overleaf as a starting point. Break your list up into food types (or order them by supermarket aisle) to make things easier when you get to the shops and alleviate your kids' pester power. Involve children in the experience and stand firm when it comes to saying no.

To avoid wastage, don't buy too much of foods that have a limited shelf life. Buy organic whenever possible, and choose seasonal fruits and vegetables. Buy a varied selection of pantry items to have on hand, and check labels and best-before dates. If you prefer not to make your own bread, wraps or rolls, opt for sourdough, brown rice or wholegrain varieties.

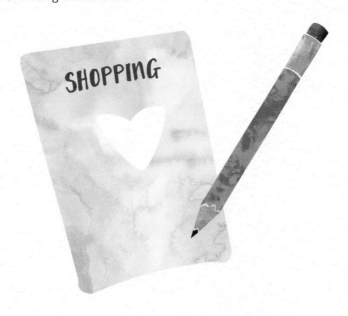

YOUR SHOPPING LIST

VEGETABLES
Bok choy (pak choy)
Broccoli
Cabbage
Capsicum (pepper)
Carrots
Cauliflower
Celery
Cherry tomatoes
Cucumber
Eggplant (aubergine)
English spinach leaves
French shallots
    (eschalots)
Garlic
Green beans
Kale
Lettuce and other
    salad greens
Onions
Parsnips
Peas
Pumpkin (squash)
Rocket (arugula)
Silverbeet (Swiss chard)
Snow peas (mangetout)
Spring onions (scallions)
Sprouts (all types)
Squash (pattypan squash)
Swede (rutabaga)
Sweet potatoes
Tomatoes
Turnips
Watercress
Zucchini (courgettes)

MEATS
(preferably organic)
Beef
Chicken
Duck
Ham, bacon, prosciutto
    (nitrate-free)
Lamb
Pork
Turkey
Veal

SEAFOOD
Anchovies
Prawns (shrimp)
Salmon (wild-caught)
Sardines
Sashimi
Scallops
Sea vegetables
Squid
Tuna

EGGS (organic)

DAIRY (full-fat,
preferably organic)
Butter
Cheddar cheese
Cream
Goat's cheese
Parmesan cheese
Plain yoghurt
    (additive-free)
Sheep's cheese

FATS AND OILS
Coconut oil (extra virgin)
Olive oil (cold-pressed
    extra virgin)
Seed and nut oils

SEEDS, NUTS AND
NUT BUTTERS
Almonds (whole,
    blanched, slivered)
Brazil nuts
Chia seeds
Flaxseeds (linseed)
Hazelnuts
Macadamias
Pecans
Pepitas (pumpkin seeds)
Pine nuts
Poppy seeds
Sesame seeds
Sunflower seeds
Tahini
Walnuts

LEGUMES (dried
or tinned)
Black beans
Cannellini beans
Chickpeas
    (garbanzo beans)
Lentils
Navy beans
Pinto beans
Split peas

GRAINS, FLOURS AND BAKING PRODUCTS

Almond meal (flour)
Amaranth
Baking powder (gluten- and additive-free)
Bicarbonate of soda (baking soda)
Brown rice, brown rice puffs and brown rice noodles
Buckwheat groats, flour and pasta
Cacao powder, nibs and butter
Coconut flakes, coconut flour and desiccated or shredded coconut
Flaxmeal (organic golden)
Gluten-free self-raising flour
Millet
Quinoa
Rice paper wrappers
Spelt
Tapioca flour (arrowroot)
Vanilla (alcohol-free extract or beans)
White rice

FRESH HERBS AND SPICES
(whole and ground)

Basil
Black peppercorns (for cracking fresh)
Cardamom
Chives
Cinnamon
Coriander (cilantro)
Cumin
Dill
Ginger
Mint
Nutmeg
Oregano
Parsley
Rosemary
Sage
Thyme

CONDIMENTS AND SWEETENERS

Apple cider vinegar
Brown rice crackers
Celtic sea salt (or Himalayan salt)
Coconut aminos, sugar and nectar
Dextrose (glucose)
Dijon mustard (sugar-free)
Dulse flakes
Rice malt syrup
Stevia drops and powder
Tamari (wheat-free)
Tomato paste
Vegetable stock (sugar- and additive-free)
Xylitol

EQUIPMENT

Iceblock (popsicle/ice lolly) moulds and sticks
Skewers
Toothpicks

MILKS AND DRINKS

Coconut milk
Cow's milk (full-fat organic)
Nut milks
Orange juice
Rice milk
Soda water

FRUITS

Apples
Apricots
Avocados
Bananas
Berries (fresh and frozen)
Citrus fruits
Dried blueberries
Dried cranberries
Nectarines
Oranges
Peaches
Pears
Plums
Watermelon

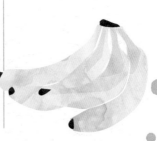

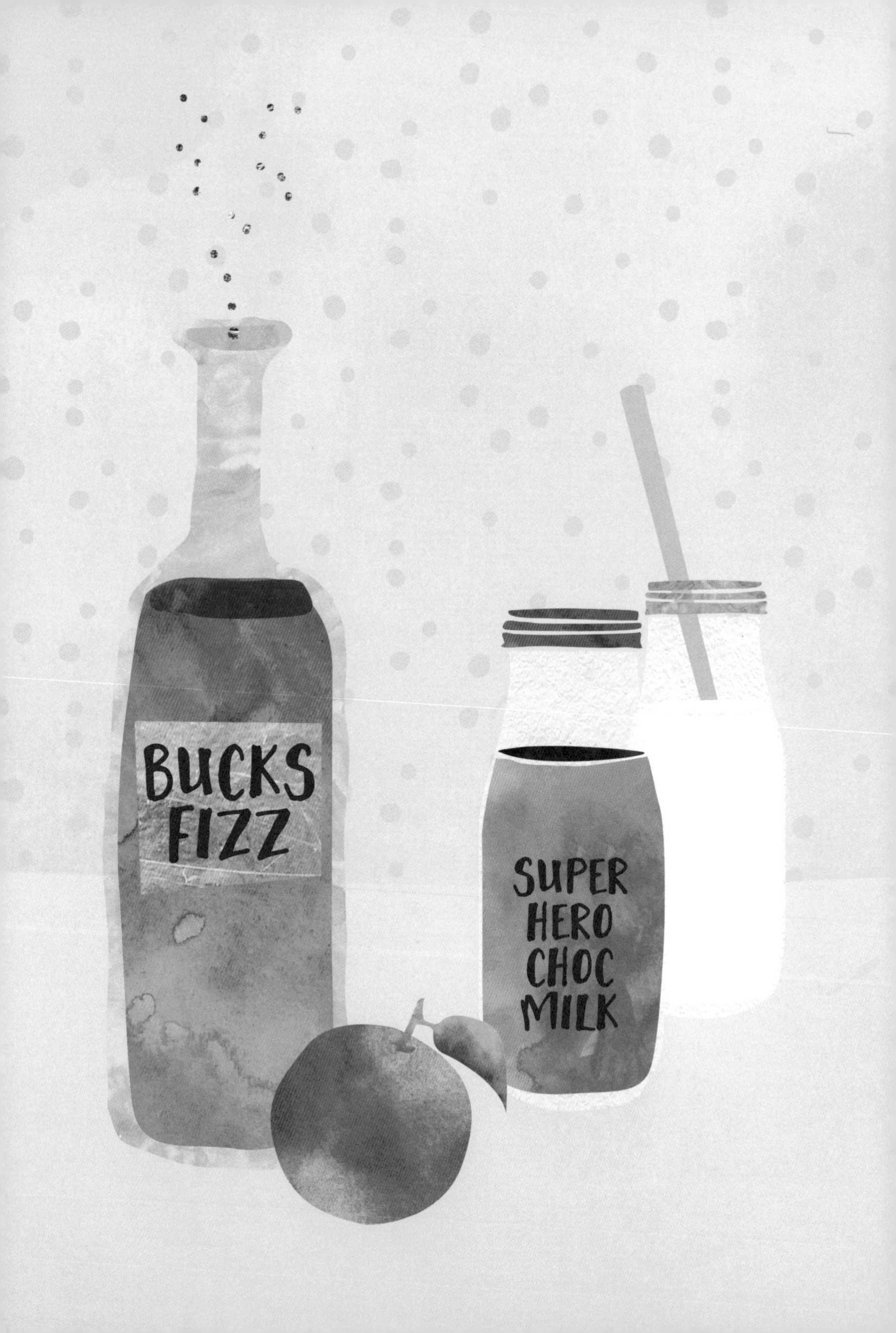
BUCKS FIZZ
SUPER HERO CHOC MILK

SHAKES AND DRINKS

From hot chocolate to cool lemonade,
the best beverages come with
a splash and dash of fun.

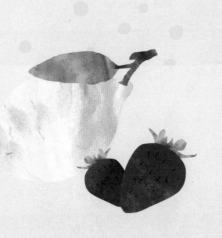

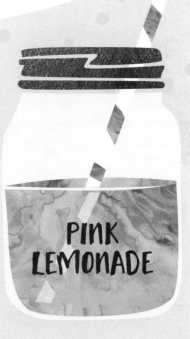

PINK
LEMONADE

SUPERHERO CHOCOLATE MILK

▲ WF ▲ DF ▲ GF ▲ VG

SERVES 2

500 ml (17 fl oz/2 cups) rice milk or nut milk
30 g (1 oz/¼ cup) cacao powder
90 g (3¼ oz/¼ cup) rice malt syrup or your sweetener of choice
½ teaspoon alcohol-free vanilla extract
135 g (4¾ oz/1 cup) ice cubes, to serve

Whizz all the ingredients in a blender until smooth. Add the ice.

 SUPERCHARGED TIP Store in a sealed container in the fridge for up to 5 days. Reheat if you feel like a warm drink.

PINK LEMONADE

▲ WF ▲ DF ▲ GF ▲ VG ▲ NF

MAKES ABOUT 1.5 LITRES (52 FL OZ/6 CUPS)

1 litre (35 fl oz/4 cups) water or sparkling water
250 ml (9 fl oz/1 cup) lemon juice (from 5–6 lemons)
1 teaspoon liquid stevia or your sweetener of choice,
    plus extra as needed
300 g (10½ oz/2 cups) fresh or frozen strawberries
ice cubes, to serve

Combine the water and lemon juice in a large jug and stir in the stevia, adding more to taste if desired. Whizz the strawberries in a food processor or blender until smooth, then add to the jug and stir to combine.

Serve over ice. If you prefer a smoother lemonade, strain before serving.

 SUPERCHARGED TIP Make a jug of this for parties instead of providing juice boxes or fizzy drinks.

BANANA AND COCONUTTY SMOOTHIE

⚠ WF ⚠ DF ⚠ GF

SERVES 2

1 banana, peeled, frozen and cut into chunks
125 ml (4 fl oz/½ cup) additive-free coconut milk
1 teaspoon ground chia seeds or flaxseed meal
1 tablespoon nut butter
130 g (4½ oz/½ cup) plain full-fat yoghurt (optional)
250 ml (9 fl oz/1 cup) almond milk or rice milk
ice cubes (optional), to serve

Whizz all the ingredients in a blender until smooth. Add ice cubes, if liked.

 SUPERCHARGED TIP This makes a great smoothie to revitalise your children after school and fill them up until dinnertime.

HEALTH TIP This creamy drink is fuelled with healthy fats, calcium and protein!

BUCKS FIZZ

⚠ WF ⚠ DF ⚠ GF ⚠ VG ⚠ NF

SERVES 2

8 fresh or frozen strawberries
250 ml (9 fl oz/1 cup) orange juice
3 ice cubes
250 ml (9 fl oz/1 cup) sparkling water

Whizz the strawberries, orange juice and ice in a blender until smooth. Pour into two cocktail glasses and add half the sparkling water to each.

VERY BERRY SHAKE

▲ WF ▲ DF ▲ GF ▲ VG

SERVES 1

125 g (4½ oz/1 cup) fresh or frozen mixed berries
½ banana, peeled and frozen
250 ml (9 fl oz/1 cup) almond milk
4 ice cubes

Whizz all the ingredients in a blender until smooth.

HEALTH TIP Need breakfast on the run? This shake will provide ample energy when time is short.

SUPERCHARGED GREEN SLUSHIE

▲ WF ▲ DF ▲ GF ▲ VG

SERVES 2

1 banana, peeled, frozen and sliced
1 tablespoon nut butter
250 ml (9 fl oz/1 cup) almond milk or rice milk
90 g (3¼ oz/2 cups) baby spinach
230 g (8 oz/1 cup) crushed ice

Whizz all the ingredients in a blender until smooth.

HEALTH TIP Sneaking in spinach will boost your child's zinc intake.

ICE CREAM SPIDER

▲ WF ▲ DF ▲ GF ▲ VG

SERVES 2

ICE CREAM
2 bananas, peeled, frozen and cut into chunks
1 tablespoon cacao powder
6 drops liquid stevia or 2 teaspoons your sweetener of choice
1 tablespoon almond butter

SODA
6 frozen raspberries, mashed
125 ml (4 fl oz/½ cup) lemon juice (from about 3 lemons)
⅛ teaspoon stevia or your sweetener of choice
250 ml (9 fl oz/1 cup) soda water or sparkling water

To prepare the ice cream, process all the ingredients in a food processor until creamy, scraping the sides as needed.

Combine the soda ingredients in a jug and stir well. If you prefer a smoother lemonade you can pass this mixture through a strainer.

Place a scoop of ice cream in each of two tall glasses and pour the soda over the top.

 SUPERCHARGED TIP Using a straw and parfait teaspoon with this drink is a lot of fun!

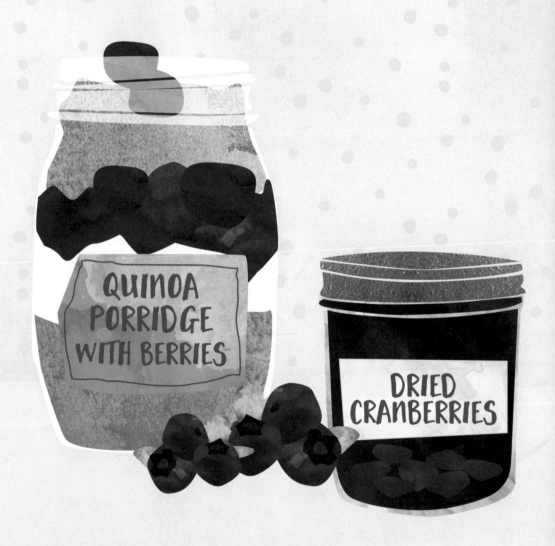

QUINOA
PORRIDGE
WITH BERRIES

DRIED
CRANBERRIES

BREAKFASTS

From brekkie-on-the-go to muffins, porridge
and jaffles, get the kids out the door in a flash.
Take the stress out of breakfast time with these
delicious and nutritious kid-friendly delights.

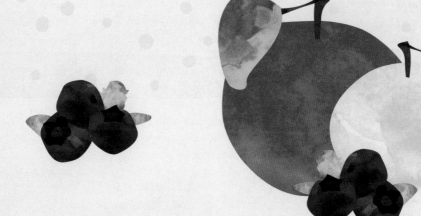

CHEESY MINI TARTLETS

▲ WF ▲ SF

MAKES 8 MINI TARTLETS

Make these ahead of time on your batch-cooking day and then just pop them in the oven to warm, or serve cold. Gluten-free filo pastry can be used for the cases if you prefer not to make your own.

PASTRY
170 g (6 oz/1²/₃ cups) almond meal
100 g (3¹/₂ oz) butter, diced, plus extra for greasing
2 tablespoons iced water

FILLING
170 ml (5¹/₂ fl oz/²/₃ cup) nut milk or rice milk
4 eggs
Celtic sea salt and freshly cracked black pepper, to taste
65 g (2¹/₄ oz/²/₃ cup) grated cheddar cheese
1 tomato, sliced

To prepare the pastry, place the almond meal in a bowl then rub in the butter with your fingers until the mixture resembles breadcrumbs. Add iced water and combine with your hands until the mixture forms a dough. Roll into a ball, wrap in plastic wrap and refrigerate for 1 hour or until firm.

Preheat the oven to 200°C (400°F) and grease eight holes of a 12 x 80 ml (2¹/₂ oz/¹/₃ cup) hole muffin tin.

Roll the pastry between two sheets of baking paper to a 30 cm x 40 cm (12 inch x 16 inch) rectangle. Cut out eight circles with a 9 cm (3¹/₂ inch) cutter and place inside the muffin tin holes. Bake for 6 minutes, then cool in the tin.

To make the filling, whisk the milk, eggs and seasoning in a bowl. Stir in the cheese, pour the mixture into the pastry cases and top each with a tomato slice. Bake for 15 minutes or until set. Cool, then remove from the pan.

 SUPERCHARGED TIP These make a great after-school snack. For a nut-free snack at recess, use gluten-free pastry.

SAVOURY BREAKFAST MUFFINS

▲ WF ▲ GF ▲ SF

MAKES 6

100 g (3½ oz/1 cup) almond meal
1 teaspoon gluten-free baking powder
½ teaspoon bicarbonate of soda (baking soda)
½ teaspoon Celtic sea salt
½ teaspoon freshly cracked black pepper
70 g (2½ oz/¼ cup) plain full-fat yoghurt
2 tablespoons butter, melted, plus extra for greasing
2 eggs
80 g (2¾ oz/½ cup) chopped additive-free ham
60 g (2¼ oz/½ cup) crumbled goat's cheese or
    50 g (1¾ oz/½ cup) grated cheddar cheese
70 g (2½ oz/½ cup) grated zucchini (courgette)
1 teaspoon finely chopped chives

Preheat the oven to 175°C (345°F) and grease a 6 x 80 ml (2½ fl oz/⅓ cup) hole muffin tin.

Combine the almond meal, baking powder, bicarbonate of soda, salt and pepper in a bowl. In a separate bowl, whisk together the yoghurt, butter and eggs. Add to the flour mixture with the remaining ingredients and use a large spoon to stir until well combined.

Spoon evenly into the muffin tin holes. Bake for 20 minutes or until golden. Cool in the tin for 10 minutes then turn out onto a wire rack to cool fully.

The muffins will keep in an airtight container in the fridge for up to 3 days. Or you can freeze them and warm them in the oven when required.

 SUPERCHARGED TIP Another delicious variation is smoked salmon. To make them lunchbox-friendly replace the almond meal with 100 g (3½ oz) of your favourite gluten-free flour.

HEALTH TIP This protein-filled muffin will start your child's day off on the right foot and provide the energy they need to get through the morning.

HOMEMADE BAKED BEANS ON TOAST

△ WF　△ DF　△ SF　△ VG　△ NF

SERVES 3

250 g (9 oz/1¼ cups) great northern beans, or your beans of choice,
　soaked overnight and drained
1 teaspoon coriander seeds
1 teaspoon fennel seeds
1 teaspoon ground turmeric
2 tablespoons extra virgin olive oil
2 garlic cloves, crushed
260 g (9¼ oz/1 cup) tomato passata (puréed tomatoes)
¼ teaspoon powdered stevia
1–2 tablespoons chopped rosemary
1 teaspoon Celtic sea salt
freshly cracked black pepper, to taste
gluten-free bread, to serve

Combine the beans, coriander, fennel and turmeric in a medium saucepan,
and add water to cover. Bring to the boil, then reduce the heat to low
and cook for 45 minutes or until the beans are soft. Drain the beans and
set aside.

Heat the olive oil in a large saucepan over low heat, then add the garlic and
cook for 1–2 minutes. Add the beans, passata, stevia and rosemary, and heat
through for 10 minutes. Season to taste. Serve on gluten-free bread.

 SUPERCHARGED TIP Freeze this dish and defrost when
you need a quick meal.

PEANUT BUTTER BANANA BREAD TRIFLE

▲ WF ▲ GF
SERVES 2

70 g (2¹/₂ oz/¹/₃ cup) no-added-sugar peanut butter
60 ml (2 fl oz/¹/₄ cup) almond milk or rice milk
2 slices Banana bread (page 128), chopped into cubes
130 g (4³/₄ oz/¹/₂ cup) plain full-fat yoghurt
1 large or 2 small bananas, sliced
handful of coconut flakes, to serve

Combine the peanut butter and milk in a small saucepan over medium heat, stirring until smooth. Add the banana bread and heat through for 1 minute. Layer the banana bread with yoghurt and banana. Sprinkle with coconut flakes.

FRENCH TOAST

▲ WF ▲ GF
SERVES 2

1 egg
60 ml (2 fl oz/¹/₄ cup) almond milk or rice milk
1 tablespoon flaxseed meal
¹/₂ teaspoon alcohol-free vanilla extract
8 drops liquid stevia or your sweetener of choice
2 slices Seeded loaf (page 125) or gluten-free bread
1 teaspoon butter, for shallow-frying
plain full-fat yoghurt and berries, to serve

In a bowl, whisk together the egg, milk, flaxseed meal, vanilla and stevia. Dip the bread in the egg mixture, coating it thoroughly. Melt the butter in a frying pan over medium heat, add the bread and cook for 3 minutes on each side or until golden brown. Serve with yoghurt and berries.

SUPERCHARGED BREAKFAST BARS

▲ WF   ▲ GF   ▲ NF*

MAKES 10 BARS

> 125 g (4½ oz/1¼ cups) almond meal, or flaxseed meal for nut-free*
> ¼ teaspoon Celtic sea salt
> ¼ teaspoon bicarbonate of soda (baking soda)
> 30 g (1 oz/½ cup) coconut flakes
> 170 g (5¾ oz/1¼ cups) mixed nuts, chopped, or
>   190 g (6¾ oz/1¼ cups) seeds, such as pepitas (pumpkin seeds)
>   and sunflower seeds, for nut-free*
> 2 tablespoons dried cranberries
> 60 g (2¼ oz) butter, melted
> 90 g (3¼ oz/¼ cup) rice malt syrup
> 1 teaspoon alcohol-free vanilla extract

Preheat the oven to 175°C (345°F) and line a 20 cm (8 inch) square baking dish or cake tin with baking paper. Combine the almond or flaxseed meal, salt, bicarbonate of soda, coconut flakes, nuts or seeds and cranberries in a large bowl, stirring well.

In another large bowl, combine the melted butter, rice malt syrup and vanilla, stirring well. Add the dry ingredients and mix well.

Press the mixture into the baking dish, pushing firmly to prevent crumbling. Bake for 20 minutes. Cut into bars in the tin, while still hot, then cool in the tin and refrigerate to firm up.

 SUPERCHARGED TIP If your school is a nut-free zone, these can't go in the lunchbox. Use the nut-free alternatives above or keep them as an after-school snack. Grind flaxseed yourself in a coffee grinder, then store it in the fridge.

HEALTH TIP Packed with good fats, zinc, dietary fibre and B vitamins, these bars make a great quick brekkie or snack.

ALMOND AND APPLE PANCAKES

▲ WF   ▲ GF

MAKES 6

100 g (3½ oz/1 cup) almond meal
1 small apple, grated
2 eggs
2–3 tablespoons butter or extra virgin coconut oil,
   plus extra for shallow-frying
3 tablespoons additive-free coconut milk
¼ teaspoon Celtic sea salt
1 teaspoon gluten-free baking powder
2 teaspoons ground cinnamon
1 teaspoon alcohol-free vanilla extract
nut milk or rice milk, as needed (optional)

Whizz the almond meal, apple, eggs, butter or coconut oil, coconut milk, salt, baking powder, cinnamon and vanilla in a food processor until smooth. For a thinner batter, add some nut or rice milk.

Melt a little butter or coconut oil in a frying pan over medium heat. When the oil is hot pour in one-sixth of the batter (about 60 ml/2 fl oz/¼ cup). When bubbles appear, turn using a spatula and cook the other side until golden. Repeat with the remaining batter.

 SUPERCHARGED TIP The batter will keep in the fridge for up to 3 days.

HEALTH TIP Full of healthy fats, vitamin E and magnesium, these pancakes will hit the spot and prepare your child for a day of learning.

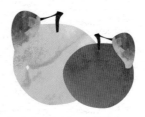

CHEESY BACON AND EGG SCRAMBLE

▲ WF   ▲ GF   ▲ SF   ▲ NF

SERVES 2

> 1 tablespoon butter
> 100 g (3½ oz/⅔ cup) chopped bacon
> 5 eggs
> 2 tablespoons water
> pinch of Celtic sea salt
> freshly cracked black pepper, to taste
> 65 g (2¼ oz/⅔ cup) grated cheddar cheese
> 2 tablespoons chopped chives

Melt the butter in a frying pan over medium heat. Add the bacon and cook for 4-5 minutes or until golden.

Whisk the eggs and water together and season with salt and pepper. Pour into the pan and stir with a fork for a few minutes to scramble. Stir through the cheese and chives, and serve.

BREAKFAST YOGHURT FRUIT COCKTAIL

▲ WF   ▲ GF

SERVES 2

> handful of Gluten-free muesli (page 64)
> 130 g (4¾ oz/½ cup) plain full-fat yoghurt
> 70 g (2½ oz/½ cup) mixed berries
> 1 tablespoon rice malt syrup or your sweetener of choice

Layer the muesli, yoghurt and berries in two glasses. Drizzle with syrup.

 SUPERCHARGED TIP Sprinkle chia seeds on the yoghurt for even more goodness. To skip the sweetener, grate some apple on top.

QUINOA PORRIDGE WITH BERRIES

WF   DF   GF   VG

SERVES 2

375 ml (13 fl oz/1½ cups) rice milk or your nut milk of choice
½ teaspoon alcohol-free vanilla extract
½ teaspoon ground cinnamon
½ teaspoon ground nutmeg
½ teaspoon ground cardamom
pinch of Celtic sea salt
100 g (3½ oz/½ cup) quinoa, rinsed and drained
8 drops liquid stevia or your sweetener of choice
your choice of berries, nuts, seeds, shredded coconut, cacao nibs,
   coconut oil or nut butter, to serve

Combine 250 ml (9 fl oz/1 cup) of the milk with the vanilla, spices and salt in a medium saucepan over medium heat and bring to the boil. Add the quinoa, then reduce the heat to low and simmer, covered, for 15 minutes.

Remove from the heat and set aside, covered, for 5 minutes. Add the stevia. Spoon into bowls and pour the remaining milk over the top. Add your topping of choice and dig in.

HEALTH TIP Quinoa is high in protein and an excellent source of magnesium and potassium.

GLUTEN-FREE MUESLI

WF ▲ DF ▲ GF ▲ VG

SERVES 6

165 g (5¾ oz/1 cup) roasted buckwheat
1 tablespoon chia seeds
55 g (2 oz/⅓ cup) sunflower seeds
80 g (2¾ oz/½ cup) almonds, chopped
½ teaspoon ground cinnamon
90 g (3¼ oz/¼ cup) rice malt syrup
15 g (½ oz/¼ cup) coconut flakes
80 g (2¾ oz/½ cup) dried fruit, such as blueberries,
   goji berries or cranberries
50 g (1¾ oz/2 cups) brown rice puffs
almond milk or rice milk, fruit and plain full-fat
   yoghurt (optional), to serve

Preheat the oven to 160°C (315°F) and line a baking tray with baking paper.

In a large bowl combine the buckwheat, chia seeds, sunflower seeds, almonds, cinnamon and rice malt syrup. Spread the mixture out on the baking tray and bake for 10 minutes, stirring occasionally. Add the coconut flakes and bake for a further 5 minutes. Cool. Add the dried fruit and rice puffs.

Serve with almond or rice milk and fresh fruit. If your child eats dairy, add a dollop of yoghurt.

 SUPERCHARGED TIP Make a big batch of this to keep on hand in your pantry.

HEALTH TIP This muesli contains just about every vitamin and mineral your child needs to keep them focused and energetic. Eat up for brain power!

CHIA COCONUT PIKELETS

▲ WF   ▲ GF   ▲ NF

MAKES 12

1 tablespoon chia seeds
210 g (7½ oz/1½ cups) self-raising gluten-free flour
250 ml (9 fl oz/1 cup) additive-free coconut milk
125 ml (4 fl oz/½ cup) water
2 eggs, beaten
1 tablespoon coconut nectar or your sweetener of choice,
    plus extra to serve
2 tablespoons butter
berries, banana and coconut flakes, to serve

Combine the chia seeds and flour in a medium bowl. In a separate bowl, whisk together the milk, water, eggs and sweetener until smooth. Gradually add the wet ingredients to the dry, whisking constantly. Set aside for 30–40 minutes or until the mixture is starting to thicken.

Heat a medium frying pan over medium heat and add a little of the butter. Pour 60 ml (2 fl oz/¼ cup) of the mixture into the pan and cook until bubbles start to form. Turn over using a spatula and cook until browned. Repeat with the remaining batter.

Serve with the extra coconut nectar, and with the berries, banana and coconut flakes.

HEALTH TIP Any time you can squeeze chia into your child's diet, you're boosting their intake of omega-3s, protein and fibre.

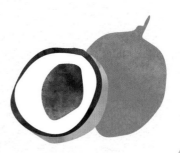

FLUFFY BANANA COCONUT PANCAKES

▲ WF ▲ DF ▲ GF ▲ NF*

MAKES 6

2 ripe bananas, plus extra, sliced, to serve
3 eggs, lightly beaten
1 tablespoon rice malt syrup, plus extra for drizzling
30 g (1 oz/¼ cup) coconut flour
¼ teaspoon Celtic sea salt
½ teaspoon bicarbonate of soda (baking soda)
1 teaspoon ground cinnamon
1 teaspoon vanilla powder
coconut oil, for shallow-frying
almond milk, or water for nut-free*, to thin, as needed
finely chopped walnuts, to serve

Mash the bananas in a bowl, then stir in the eggs and rice malt syrup. Combine the dry ingredients in a separate bowl, then add to the banana mixture and stir to combine. Whizz the mixture in a blender on high for 1 minute.

Melt the coconut oil in a frying pan over medium heat. Add 60 ml (2 fl oz/ ¼ cup) batter to the pan. (If the batter is too thick, add a little almond milk or water.) Cook for 5–6 minutes or until golden and set, then turn over and cook for 1–2 minutes on the other side. Repeat with the remaining batter.

Stack the pancakes on a plate, top with sliced banana and walnuts, and drizzle with extra rice malt syrup.

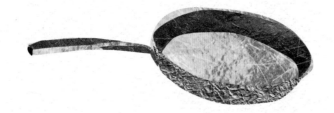

TOMATO AND QUINOA MUFFINS

⚠ WF ⚠ GF ⚠ SF ⚠ NF

MAKES 12

> 880 g (1 lb 15 oz/4 cups) cooked quinoa
>   (from 220 g/7³/₄ oz uncooked quinoa)
> 2 eggs
> 1 onion, finely chopped
> 120 g (4¼ oz/1 cup) goat's cheese, or 100 g (3½ oz/1 cup)
>   grated cheddar cheese
> large handful of coriander (cilantro), finely chopped
> 45 g (1½ oz/⅓ cup) cherry tomatoes, chopped
> ½ teaspoon Celtic sea salt
> ½ teaspoon freshly cracked black pepper

Preheat the oven to 175°C (345°F) and line a 12 x 80 ml (2½ oz/⅓ cup) hole muffin tin with paper cases.

Combine all the ingredients in a large bowl and stir well. Spoon into the prepared muffin tin and smooth the tops with a spatula. Bake for 20 minutes or until golden brown. Cool in the tin for 15 minutes.

 SUPERCHARGED TIP These muffins are especially delicious when served warm. Serve with a Banana and coconutty smoothie (page 51) for a well-rounded breakfast giving long-lasting energy.

HEALTH TIP Full of protein, these are a great energy-boosting breakfast for busy kids.

BLUEBERRY AND COCONUT MUFFINS

△ WF   △ GF

MAKES 6

250 ml (9 fl oz/1 cup) almond milk or rice milk
40 g (1½ oz/¼ cup) chia seeds
120 g (4¼ oz/1 cup) coconut flour
½ teaspoon bicarbonate of soda (baking soda)
½ teaspoon gluten-free baking powder
¼ teaspoon Celtic sea salt
1 teaspoon alcohol-free vanilla extract
140 g (5 oz/1 cup) coconut sugar
5 eggs
125 g (4½ oz) butter, melted
155 g (5½ oz/1 cup) blueberries (fresh or frozen)

Preheat the oven to 175°C (345°F) and line a 6 x 250 ml (9 fl oz/1 cup) hole muffin tin with paper cases. Mix half the milk with the chia seeds and set aside for 30 minutes.

Combine the coconut flour, bicarbonate of soda, baking powder, salt, vanilla and coconut sugar in a large bowl. In a separate bowl, whisk together the eggs, melted butter and remaining milk, then stir in the blueberries and chia mix.

Add to the dry mix and stir to combine. Divide the mixture between the prepared muffin holes and bake for 35 minutes or until a skewer inserted into the centre of a muffin comes out clean.

 SUPERCHARGED TIP You can mix it up by changing the fruit you toss into this mix. Fresh bananas or raspberries work well, too.

HEALTH TIP These muffins are full of magnesium and omega-3s for healthy brain function.

GOAT'S CHEESE AND TOMATO JAFFLES

▲ WF ▲ GF ▲ SF

SERVES 2

> butter, for spreading
> 4 slices Seeded loaf (page 125)
> 60 g (2¼ oz/½ cup) goat's cheese
> 1 tomato, sliced

Preheat a jaffle iron or sandwich toaster. Butter one side of each slice of bread and place two slices, butter side down, on the jaffle iron or toaster. Place half the goat's cheese and tomato on each, then cover with the remaining slices of bread, butter side up. Toast the sandwich for 5 minutes or until golden.

HEALTH TIP Just by replacing traditional bread with Seeded loaf, you've boosted the nutritional benefits of this jaffle. Topped with warm, melted goat's cheese, it's a match made in heaven.

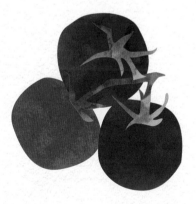

COCONUT MILK

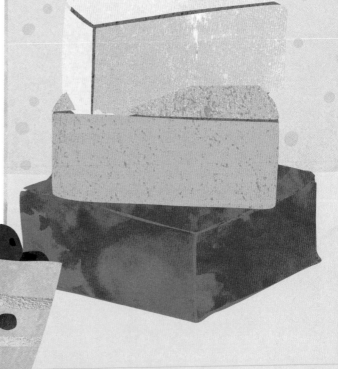

CHEDDAR CHEESE

BEFORE- AND AFTER-SCHOOL SNACKS

These nutritious snacks will get them
through the day at full speed.

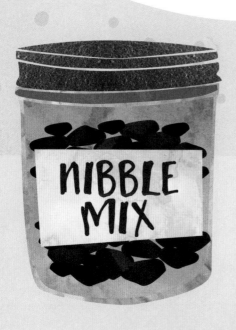

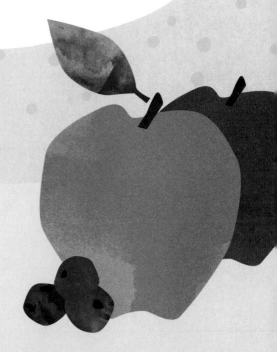

GINGERBREAD MEN

▲ WF   ▲ DF   ▲ GF

MAKES ABOUT 8

150 g (5$\frac{1}{2}$ oz/1$\frac{1}{2}$ cups) almond meal
1$\frac{1}{2}$ teaspoons stevia powder
$\frac{1}{4}$ teaspoon Celtic sea salt
3 teaspoons ground ginger
$\frac{1}{4}$ teaspoon ground nutmeg
$\frac{1}{2}$ teaspoon ground cinnamon
1 teaspoon ground cloves
1 teaspoon soda water
250 g (9 oz/1 cup) almond butter
4 eggs, lightly beaten
1 teaspoon alcohol-free vanilla extract
dried currants, to decorate (optional)

FROSTING
1 teaspoon alcohol-free vanilla extract
110 g (3$\frac{3}{4}$ oz) extra virgin coconut oil, melted
80 ml (2$\frac{1}{2}$ fl oz/$\frac{1}{3}$ cup) coconut nectar or 120 g (4$\frac{1}{4}$ oz/$\frac{1}{3}$ cup)
  rice malt syrup or your sweetener of choice
80 ml (2$\frac{1}{2}$ fl oz/$\frac{1}{3}$ cup) additive-free coconut milk
pinch of Celtic sea salt

Preheat the oven to 175°C (345°F) and line a baking tray with baking paper.

Combine the almond meal, stevia, salt, spices and soda water in a large
bowl and stir well. Warm the almond butter in a bowl resting on a saucepan
of boiling water on the stovetop, ensuring the bowl does not touch the
water. Add the eggs and vanilla, and whisk until the mixture is smooth.
Add to the almond meal mixture and mix well.

Roll the mixture to 5 mm ($\frac{1}{4}$ inch) thickness and use a gingerbread man
cutter to cut out shapes. Place on the prepared baking tray, leaving space
between them to allow for spreading. Decorate with currants or draw on
a design with a toothpick.

Bake for 15–20 minutes or until crisp and golden. Cool a little on the tray before transferring to a wire rack to cool completely.

To make the frosting, whizz all the ingredients in a blender until combined. Pour into a bowl and refrigerate for 15 minutes, then blend again. Use to decorate the biscuits, then refrigerate to harden further if required.

 SUPERCHARGED TIP Almond meal and almond flour are the same thing and can be used interchangeably. Blend the frosting with raspberries or blueberries to create a colourful icing the kids will love.

HEALTH TIP Almonds are full of nutrients that aid brain development.

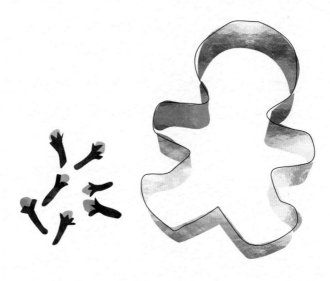

NIBBLE MIX

▲ WF ▲ DF ▲ GF ▲ SF ▲ VG
MAKES 4 CUPS

160 g (5½ oz/1 cup) almonds
155 g (5½ oz/1 cup) cashews
75 g (2½ oz/½ cup) pepitas (pumpkin seeds)
75 g (2½ oz/½ cup) sunflower seeds
125 ml (4 fl oz/½ cup) wheat-free tamari
90 g (3¼ oz) brown rice crackers, broken into bite-sized pieces

Preheat the oven to 160°C (315°F) and line a baking tray with baking paper.

Combine all the ingredients except the rice crackers in a bowl, stirring to coat all the nuts and seeds with the tamari. Spoon onto the prepared baking tray and bake for 25 minutes. Cool, then add the rice crackers. Store in an airtight container until ready to eat.

 SUPERCHARGED TIP Pepitas should be green. If they're brown, it can indicate that they're rancid.

HEALTH TIP Full of zinc, protein and vitamins B and E, this is the perfect after-school snack to boost energy and allay the pre-dinner hunger pangs.

PROSCIUTTO ROLL-UPS

▲ WF ▲ GF ▲ NF
SERVES 2

1 green apple
30 g (1 oz/¼ cup) goat's cheese
4 slices prosciutto

Cut the apple into quarters then slice thinly. Spread a thin layer of goat's cheese on each piece of prosciutto, top with an apple slice and roll up!

SWEET AND SOUR POTATO FRIES WITH APPLE CIDER VINEGAR

▲ WF   ▲ DF   ▲ GF   ▲ SF   ▲ VG   ▲ NF

SERVES 3

2 teaspoons extra virgin olive oil
2 tablespoons apple cider vinegar
Celtic sea salt, to taste
2 sweet potatoes, peeled and cut into fries

Preheat the oven to 175°C (345°C) and line a baking tray with baking paper.

Mix the olive oil, apple cider vinegar and salt in a bowl. Add the sweet potato and toss to coat well.

Arrange in a single layer on the prepared tray and bake for 30 minutes or until golden and cooked through.

 SUPERCHARGED TIP These yummy sweet-and-sour fries are healthier than regular French fries and taste great with a dip (see pages 98–101).

HEALTH TIP Sweet potatoes have a much lower GI than white potatoes and are a great source of vitamin B, vitamin C and magnesium.

CACAO BOMB CRACKLES

WF   DF   GF   VG   NF

MAKES 12

70 g (2½ oz / ½ cup) coconut sugar
110 g (3¾ oz / ½ cup) extra virgin coconut oil
2 tablespoons coconut butter
30 g (1 oz / ¼ cup) cacao powder
1 teaspoon alcohol-free vanilla extract
45 g (1½ oz / ½ cup) desiccated coconut
50 g (1¾ oz / 2 cups) brown rice puffs

Line a 12 x 80 ml (2½ fl oz / ⅓ cup) hole muffin tin with paper cases.

Process the coconut sugar to a fine powder in a food processor. Place a bowl over a saucepan of boiling water over medium heat, ensuring the bowl does not touch the water. Add the coconut sugar, coconut oil, coconut butter, cacao powder and vanilla, then stir until melted and combined.

Remove from the heat, add the desiccated coconut and rice puffs, and stir well. Spoon into the prepared muffin tin and refrigerate until set.

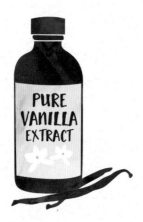

NUT BUTTER STARS

WF　　DF　　GF

MAKES ABOUT 36 STARS (DEPENDING ON SIZE OF CUTTER)

> 1 large egg
> 105 g (3½ oz/¾ cup) coconut sugar
> 1 teaspoon bicarbonate of soda (baking soda)
> ½ teaspoon alcohol-free vanilla extract
> 250 g (9 oz/1 cup) nut butter
> gluten-free plain (all-purpose) flour, for dusting

Preheat the oven to 175°C (345°F) and line two baking trays with baking paper.

Beat the egg, coconut sugar, bicarbonate of soda and vanilla using an electric mixer. Add the nut butter and beat to combine. Keep beating until the mixture thickens to a dough-like consistency.

On a floured bench, roll out the mixture to 4 mm (³/₁₆ inch) thickness and use a star cutter to cut out shapes. Place on the prepared baking trays and bake for 10 minutes or until just set. Cool on the trays for 5–10 minutes then transfer to a wire rack to cool completely.

 SUPERCHARGED TIP You can cut these into any shape you like! If you don't have a cookie cutter, just use a knife to cut out squares or circles (an upside-down glass is good for this, too).

HEALTH TIP These biscuits are much healthier than the packaged ones you find in a supermarket. Making your own biscuits means you can control the ingredients and avoid anything artificial.

4 PM PICK-UP BICKS

▲ WF   ▲ GF   ▲ SF

MAKES 12–16

100 g (3¹/₂ oz/1 cup) almond meal, plus extra for dusting
pinch of Celtic sea salt
90 g (3¹/₄ oz) unsalted butter, chilled
225 g (8 oz/2¹/₄ cups) grated cheddar cheese
60–80 ml (2–2¹/₂ fl oz/¹/₄–¹/₃ cup) iced water

Combine the almond meal, salt and butter in a food processor until the mixture resembles breadcrumbs. Add the cheese and pulse to combine. With the motor running, slowly add the water until the mixture forms a dough. Wrap the dough in plastic wrap and refrigerate for 30 minutes.

Preheat the oven to 175°C (345°F) and line a baking tray with baking paper.

Roll the dough on a lightly floured bench to 1 cm (¹/₂ inch) thickness. Cut into small squares with a knife, then use a fork to prick the biscuits to make a pattern. Using a palette knife, transfer the squares to the prepared baking tray. Bake for 15 minutes or until golden.

SUPERCHARGED TIP Serve with slices of stone fruit and a Crunchy chicken drummer (page 105) for a well-rounded, nutritionally dense snack or meal.

CUCUMBER SAILING BOATS

▲ WF   ▲ GF   ▲ SF

SERVES 2

2 small Lebanese (short) cucumbers
260 g (9¼ oz/1 cup) plain full-fat yoghurt
6 drops liquid stevia or 2 teaspoons your sweetener of choice
pinch of Celtic sea salt
1 tablespoon chopped dill
1 red capsicum (pepper), seeded
toothpicks, for decorating

Cut the cucumbers in half lengthways and scoop out the seeds.

Combine the yoghurt, stevia, salt and dill in a bowl. Spoon into the hollowed-out cucumbers.

Cut triangles for sails out of the capsicum. Skewer each sail with a toothpick and stick the other end in the cucumber.

 SUPERCHARGED TIP This is a great snack to let the kids make on their own – with parental supervision.

HEALTH TIP Cucumbers are mostly water, so they're a great way to keep the body hydrated. They're also a good source of B vitamins, so they'll give your child a little energy boost.

CELERY AND CARROTS WITH NUT BUTTER DIPPING SAUCE

▲ WF ▲ DF ▲ GF ▲ SF ▲ VG ▲ NF*

SERVES 3

2 carrots, cut into sticks
2 celery stalks, cut into batons

DIPPING SAUCE
3 tablespoons nut butter, or seed butter for nut-free*
6 drops liquid stevia or 2 teaspoons your sweetener of choice
1 tablespoon wheat-free tamari
4 drops sesame oil

Combine all the dipping sauce ingredients in a bowl and whisk well.
For a thinner dip, add a little water.

Serve with the carrot and celery sticks.

 SUPERCHARGED TIP Send this dip to school for lunch by storing it in an airtight plastic container. Add some Seeded loaf (page 125) for a well-rounded meal. If your school is a nut-free zone, make sure you use seed butter rather than nut butter in the dipping sauce.

HEALTH TIP Full of vitamins and antioxidants, this meal is one easy way to boost your child's vegie intake.

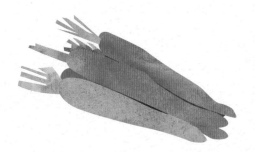

NUTTY CHOCOLATE BISCUITS

▲ WF ▲ GF

MAKES 12

Kids will love these delicious melt-in-the-mouth biscuits after school.

> 250 g (9 oz/2½ cups) almond meal
> 55 g (2 oz/½ cup) cacao powder
> ½ teaspoon Celtic sea salt
> ½ teaspoon bicarbonate of soda (baking soda)
> 125 g (4½ oz) butter, melted
> 180 g (6¼ oz/½ cup) rice malt syrup
> 1 teaspoon alcohol-free vanilla extract
> 2 tablespoons cacao nibs
> 65 g (2¼ oz/½ cup) slivered almonds

Preheat the oven to 175°C (345°F) and line a baking tray with baking paper.

Combine the almond meal, cacao powder, salt and bicarbonate of soda in a large bowl. In a separate bowl combine the melted butter, rice malt syrup and vanilla. Add the wet ingredients to the dry and mix well. Stir through the cacao nibs and almonds.

Spoon tablespoons of dough onto the prepared baking tray and flatten using a spatula. Bake for 8 minutes then cool on the trays.

ORANGE AND CRANBERRY MUFFINS

WF GF NF

MAKES 6

60 g (2¼ oz/½ cup) coconut flour
1 teaspoon gluten-free baking powder
½ teaspoon bicarbonate of soda (baking soda)
grated zest of 1 orange, plus 2 tablespoons orange juice
75 g (2½ oz/½ cup) dried cranberries
1 teaspoon powdered stevia or your sweetener of choice
4 eggs, lightly beaten
⅛ teaspoon alcohol-free vanilla extract or orange extract
60 g (2¼ oz) butter, melted
125 ml (4 fl oz/½ cup) additive-free coconut milk

Preheat the oven to 180°C (350°F) and grease a 6 x 250 ml (9 fl oz/1 cup) hole muffin tin.

Combine the flour, baking powder, bicarbonate of soda, orange zest, cranberries and stevia in a bowl and mix well. In a separate bowl, combine the orange juice, eggs, vanilla, butter and coconut milk. Add the dry ingredients to the wet and mix well.

Spoon the mixture into the prepared muffin tin and bake for 18–20 minutes or until golden and firm. Cool on a wire rack.

 SUPERCHARGED TIP When baking with coconut flour, you need to increase the number of eggs to achieve a delicious, moist cake. These muffins can be made dairy-free by replacing the butter with mild olive oil.

HEALTH TIP Kids love a little cake, and these are full of healthy protein and fibre as well as lauric acid, which helps boost the immune system.

PIRATE MUESLI BARS

▲ WF   ▲ DF   ▲ GF   ▲ VG

MAKES ABOUT 12 BARS

> 55 g (2 oz) extra virgin coconut oil, or 60 g (2¼ oz) butter
> 120 g (4¼ oz/⅓ cup) rice malt syrup or your sweetener of choice
> 2 teaspoons alcohol-free vanilla extract
> pinch of Celtic sea salt
> 280 g (10 oz/2 cups) mixed seeds, such as pepitas (pumpkin seeds)
>   or sesame, sunflower or chia seeds
> 65 g (2¼ oz/¾ cup) desiccated coconut

Preheat the oven to 150°C (300°F) and line an 18 cm (7 inch) square cake tin with baking paper.

Melt the coconut oil or butter in a medium saucepan over medium heat. Add the rice malt syrup, vanilla and salt, and stir until combined. Remove from the heat and stir in the seeds and coconut.

Spoon the mixture into the prepared cake tin and press down firmly. Bake for 10 minutes, then cool on a wire rack. Chill in the fridge then cut into bars.

 SUPERCHARGED TIP Muesli bars are an easy snack to drop into the lunchbox. Homemade muesli bars are much healthier and just as yummy.

HEALTH TIP This seed-filled bar is packed with vitamins, selenium and antioxidants – all crucial in fighting disease and preventing cellular damage.

ZOO POO

WF   DF   GF   SF   VG   NF*
MAKES 8

60 g (2¼ oz) coconut butter
2 teaspoons stevia powder
1 tablespoon cacao powder
80 ml (2½ fl oz/⅓ cup) almond milk, or rice milk for nut-free*
30 g (1 oz/½ cup) coconut flakes

Melt the coconut butter in a bowl over a saucepan of boiling water,
ensuring the bowl does not touch the water. Stir through the stevia and
cacao until smooth. Remove from the heat, add the milk and stir until
thickened. Take 1 tablespoon of the mixture at a time and roll into balls.
Roll in the coconut flakes and place on a tray. Refrigerate until set.

HEALTH TIP Cacao powder is loaded with antioxidants and
although sometimes bitter, it can be made sweeter with the
addition of a natural sweetener.

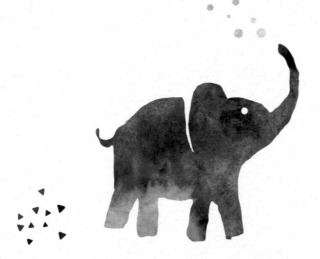

CHICKEN NUGGETS

▲ WF ◢ DF ▲ GF ▲ SF

SERVES 3

100 g (3½ oz/1 cup) almond meal
pinch of Celtic sea salt
freshly cracked black pepper or lemon pepper, to taste
2 chicken breast fillets, cut into nugget-sized pieces
3 eggs, lightly beaten
70 g (2½ oz) coconut oil, for shallow-frying

Mix the almond meal and seasonings together. Dip the chicken in the egg, then roll in the almond mix.

Melt the coconut oil in a frying pan over medium–high heat. Add the chicken and cook until golden brown on both sides.

Serve with a dip of your choice (see pages 98–101).

 SUPERCHARGED TIP You can include ground flaxseeds with the almond meal in this recipe for an extra nutrient burst.

HEALTH TIP Coconut oil contains good fats that promote heart health and low cholesterol.

MINI SPRING ROLLS

▲ WF   ▲ DF   ▲ GF   ▲ SF   ▲ VG   ▲ NF

MAKES 8–10

2 teaspoons coconut oil, plus extra for shallow-frying
1 carrot, thinly sliced
1 zucchini (courgette), thinly sliced
¼ butternut pumpkin (squash), seeded and cut into thin strips
¼ red cabbage, shredded
1 small onion, thinly sliced
8–10 x 15 cm (6 inch) rice paper wrappers

Melt the coconut oil in a large frying pan over medium–high heat, then add the vegetables and cook, stirring frequently, for 5–7 minutes or until softened. Set aside to cool.

Soften the rice paper wrappers in water following the packet instructions. Place a wrapper on a clean surface, then take a small handful of the vegetable mixture and place it in the centre. Fold in the sides and roll up from the bottom. Repeat with the remaining wrappers and mixture.

Heat some coconut oil in a non-stick frying pan over medium heat and fry the rolls, two at a time, being careful to keep them separated and turning them to brown all over. Remove from the frying pan and rest on a baking tray to cool. (Alternatively, brush the rolls with melted coconut oil and bake in a 180°C/350°F oven for 20 minutes or until cooked through.) Serve with a dipping sauce (see pages 80 and 100).

SEASONED WINGS

▲ WF ▲ DF ▲ GF ▲ SF ▲ NF
SERVES 3

125 ml (4 fl oz/ 1/2 cup) apple cider vinegar
60 ml (2 fl oz/ 1/4 cup) extra virgin olive oil
2 tablespoons wheat-free tamari
6 drops liquid stevia
1 egg, lightly beaten
1/2 teaspoon Celtic sea salt
freshly cracked black pepper, to taste
6 chicken wings

Preheat the oven to 175°C (345°F).

In a large bowl, mix the vinegar, oil, tamari, stevia, egg, salt and pepper. Add the chicken wings to the bowl, and stir to ensure they're covered in the marinade. Cover and refrigerate for 1 hour.

Arrange the chicken wings in a baking dish and pour over one-quarter of the marinade mixture. Bake for 30 minutes. Pour off any liquid and return to the oven for another 5 minutes, or until the chicken is cooked through.

 SUPERCHARGED TIP Serve with Apple Slaw (page 94).

HEALTH TIP Apple cider vinegar helps your body regulate its pH and can help stimulate blood circulation.

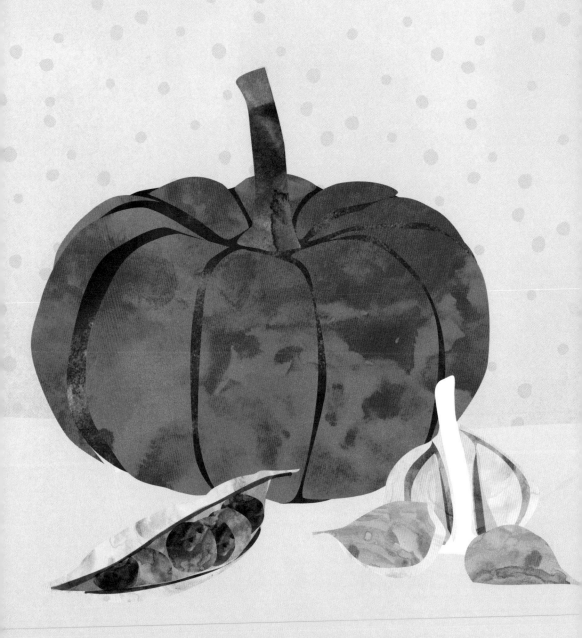

SOUPS AND SALADS

Why choose one or the other? Serve a small cup of soup with a side serving of salad to create a nutritionally balanced meal fit for your prince or princess.

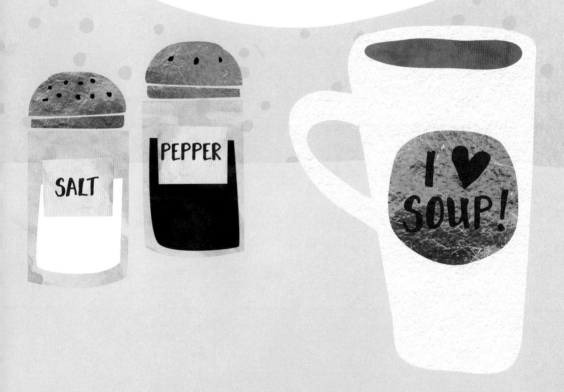

SALT

PEPPER

I ♥ SOUP!

PEA, HAM AND MINT SOUP

▲ WF ▲ DF ▲ GF ▲ SF ▲ NF

SERVES 4

1 tablespoon extra virgin olive oil
1 onion, chopped
2 garlic cloves, crushed
2 celery stalks, thinly sliced, plus small handful of leaves, torn
440 g (15½ oz/2 cups) green split peas, rinsed and drained
1.5 litres (52 fl oz/6 cups) chicken stock
1 tablespoon lemon juice
250 g (9 oz) sliced leg ham, chopped
small handful of mint leaves, torn

Heat the olive oil in a large saucepan over low-medium heat. Add the onion, garlic and celery, and cook, stirring frequently, for 3-4 minutes or until the onion is translucent.

Add the peas, stock and lemon juice, then cover, increase the heat to high and bring to the boil. Reduce the heat to medium and simmer, partially covered, for 30 minutes or until the peas are tender but not mushy.

Stir in the ham, mint and celery leaves, and cook, stirring frequently, for 2 minutes. Dish it up and enjoy.

 SUPERCHARGED TIP Make a big batch of soup and freeze it for a busy weeknight meal when you're running short of time.

CREAMY PUMPKIN SOUP

▲ WF   ▲ DF   ▲ GF   ▲ SF   ▲ VG   ▲ NF

SERVES 3

2 tablespoons extra virgin olive oil
1 onion, diced
1 butternut pumpkin (squash), peeled, seeded and diced
1 small sweet potato, peeled and diced
1 carrot, peeled and roughly chopped
500 ml (17 fl oz/2 cups) vegetable stock or water
270 ml (9½ fl oz) tin additive-free coconut milk
Celtic sea salt and freshly cracked black pepper, to taste

Heat the olive oil in a large saucepan over medium heat. Add the onion and cook for 3–4 minutes or until softened. Add the vegetables and cook for 6–7 minutes or until golden.

Add the stock and bring to the boil. Reduce the heat to low and simmer, covered, for 20 minutes or until the vegetables are soft. Add the coconut milk and cook for a further 2 minutes.

Allow to cool slightly, then purée in a blender or food processor until smooth. Season with salt and pepper.

HEALTH TIP Pumpkin is full of carotenoids, which help prevent disease. It's also a natural source of vitamin A, which can boost the immune system.

CHICKEN NOODLE SOUP

WF   DF   GF   SF   NF

SERVES 4

250 g (9 oz) brown rice noodles or zucchini noodles
  made from 3 zucchini (courgettes)
1 tablespoon coconut oil
1 onion, chopped
2 chicken breasts, roughly chopped
3 celery stalks, sliced, plus 4 leaves, torn
1 carrot, sliced
½ teaspoon thyme leaves
1 teaspoon dried parsley
Celtic sea salt and freshly cracked black pepper, to taste
1.5 litres (52 fl oz/6 cups) chicken stock
1 tablespoon wheat-free tamari
1 tablespoon apple cider vinegar
2 bay leaves

Cook the noodles until al dente according to the packet directions. (If using zucchini noodles, leave them raw.)

Heat the coconut oil in a medium saucepan over medium heat. Add the onion and cook for 3–4 minutes or until translucent. Add the chicken and cook for 4 minutes, stirring frequently. Add the celery stalks and leaves, carrot, thyme and parsley, and cook for a further 3 minutes. Season with salt and pepper.

Add the stock, tamari, apple cider vinegar and bay leaves. Bring to the boil then reduce the heat and simmer for 20 minutes.

Just before serving the soup, add the noodles and stir to separate. Adjust the seasoning and serve.

JOLLY GREEN GIANT SOUP

▲ WF   ▲ DF   ▲ GF   ▲ SF   ▲ VG   ▲ NF

SERVES 4

1 tablespoon extra virgin olive oil
2 cups mixed vegetables, such as zucchini (courgette),
    cucumber, lettuce, English spinach, celery and broccoli
500 ml (17 fl oz/2 cups) vegetable stock or water
250 ml (9 fl oz/1 cup) additive-free coconut milk
freshly grated nutmeg, to taste
Celtic sea salt and freshly cracked black pepper, to taste

Heat the olive oil in a medium saucepan over medium heat. Add the
vegetables and cook, stirring frequently, for 4–5 minutes or until starting
to soften.

Add the stock and coconut milk, and bring to the boil, then reduce the
heat and simmer until the vegetables are soft (the cooking time will vary
depending on the vegetables selected).

Remove from the heat, cool slightly, then whizz in a blender or food
processor until smooth. Add the nutmeg and season to taste.

HEALTH TIP Dark leafy greens are one of the best sources of iron,
calcium, potassium and magnesium. This is an easy and yummy way
to sneak them in!

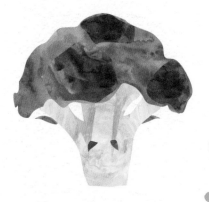

APPLE SLAW

▲ WF ◢ DF ▲ GF ▲ VG ▲ NF

SERVES 2–3

DRESSING
60 ml (2 fl oz/¼ cup) additive-free coconut milk
1 tablespoon tahini
60 ml (2 fl oz/¼ cup) lemon juice
1 teaspoon mustard
1 tablespoon chopped flat-leaf (Italian) parsley
1 tablespoon chopped mint
6 drops liquid stevia or 2 teaspoons your sweetener of choice
Celtic sea salt and freshly cracked black pepper, to taste

SLAW
2 green apples, coarsely grated or shredded
  with a mandoline
¼ red cabbage, shredded
¼ green cabbage, shredded

Combine the dressing ingredients in a large bowl and whisk until smooth. Add the apple and cabbage to the dressing and stir to coat. Adjust the seasoning. Chill before serving.

HEALTH TIP Tahini is rich in magnesium and potassium, both of which aid in promoting a calm mind and energetic learning.

QUINOA WITH CHICKPEAS AND CUCUMBER

▲ WF ▲ GF ▲ SF

SERVES 2–3

80 ml (2$\frac{1}{2}$ fl oz/$\frac{1}{3}$ cup) extra virgin olive oil
1 French shallot (eschalot), finely chopped
2 tablespoons apple cider vinegar
Celtic sea salt and freshly cracked black pepper, to taste
440 g (15$\frac{1}{2}$ oz/2 cups) cooked quinoa (from 110 g/3$\frac{3}{4}$ oz uncooked quinoa)
2 large tomatoes, diced
1 small Lebanese (short) cucumber, diced
15 g ($\frac{1}{2}$ oz/$\frac{1}{4}$ cup) chopped mint
400 g (14 oz) tin chickpeas, rinsed and drained
60 g (2$\frac{1}{4}$ oz/$\frac{1}{2}$ cup) goat's cheese

Combine the olive oil, shallot, apple cider vinegar and salt and pepper in a jar, and shake well. Combine the remaining ingredients in a large bowl, then add the dressing and stir through gently.

 SUPERCHARGED TIP Pack this for lunch as it is or use it to fill a wrap and create a scrumptious meal your child will enjoy.

HEALTH TIP High in protein and low in fat, this salad will boost energy levels without the afternoon slump.

SWEET POTATO AND APPLE SALAD

▲ WF ▲ DF ▲ GF ▲ VG

SERVES 4

DRESSING
65 g (2¼ oz/ ¼ cup) almond butter
1 tablespoon apple cider vinegar
1 tablespoon sesame oil
1 tablespoon lime juice
7 drops liquid stevia or 1 tablespoon your sweetener of choice

SALAD
1 small sweet potato, peeled and finely chopped
  (can be cooked if preferred)
1 apple, cored and finely chopped
1 celery stalk, thinly sliced
2 tablespoons sesame seeds, toasted
large handful of coriander (cilantro) leaves

Whisk the dressing ingredients together in a bowl. Combine the salad ingredients in a large bowl and drizzle with the dressing.

 SUPERCHARGED TIP Serve any of these salads as a snack or a meal – just reduce or increase the portion size to suit.

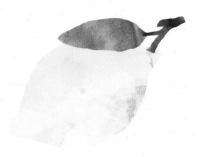

CHICKEN AND MANGO SALAD

WF   DF   GF   NF

SERVES 4

90 g (3¼ oz) baby spinach leaves
1 red capsicum (pepper), seeded and sliced
1 red onion, sliced (optional)
250 g (9 oz) cherry tomatoes, cut in half
4 chicken breasts, pan-fried and sliced
2 fresh mangoes, peeled and sliced
235 g (8½ oz/1 cup) whole egg mayonnaise

Toss the spinach, capsicum, onion (if using) and tomatoes in a bowl. Divide between serving plates and top with the chicken and mango. Drizzle with mayonnaise and serve.

TUNA AND EGG SALAD

WF   DF   GF   SF   NF

SERVES 2

185 g (6½ oz) tin tuna in extra virgin olive oil
110 g (3¾ oz/½ cup) Hummus the hero (page 101)
1 boiled egg, chopped
¼ red onion, finely chopped
2.5 cm (1 inch) piece of celery, finely chopped
1 tablespoon lemon juice
Celtic sea salt, to taste

Combine all the ingredients and serve chilled.

HEALTH TIP Tuna and egg provide a protein hit your kids will need if they're running around all day.

SIX DIPS TO TRANSFORM FUSSY EATERS

Dips are the perfect way to boost your child's vegie intake while making the meal fun and interactive. No complaints!

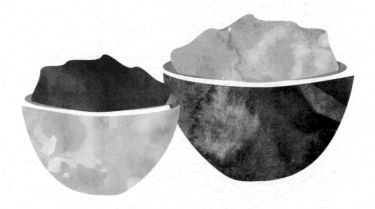

1 SALSA DIP

▲ WF ▲ DF ▲ GF ▲ SF ▲ VG ▲ NF

MAKES 375 ML (13 FL OZ/1½ CUPS)

3 tomatoes, chopped
60 g (2¼ oz/½ cup) chopped spring onion (scallion)
80 g (2¾ oz/½ cup) green capsicum (pepper), diced
large handful of coriander (cilantro) leaves
juice of 1 lime
1 teaspoon Celtic sea salt

Combine all the ingredients in a bowl and mix gently.

 SUPERCHARGED TIP Serve this dip (and the others) with 4 pm Pick-up bicks (page 78), rice or gluten-free crackers, and carrot, celery, cucumber and capsicum (pepper) sticks.

---

2 CUCUMBER AND YOGHURT DIP

▲ WF ▲ GF ▲ SF ▲ NF

MAKES 375 ML (13 FL OZ/1½ CUPS)

1 medium Lebanese (short) cucumber, peeled, cut in half
   lengthways, seeds removed
260 g (9¼ oz/1 cup) plain full-fat yoghurt
1 garlic clove, crushed
1 teaspoon ground cumin
large handful of mint leaves, finely chopped
Celtic sea salt, to taste

Grate the cucumber using the large-holed side of a grater. Transfer to a sieve and squeeze the liquid out with your hands. Combine with the remaining ingredients in a medium bowl and stir well.

3 ASIAN DIPPING SAUCE

▲ WF ▲ DF ▲ GF ▲ SF ▲ VG

MAKES 125 ML (4 FL OZ/ ½ CUP)

2 tablespoons wheat-free tamari, plus extra to taste
2 teaspoons sesame oil
6 drops liquid stevia or 2 teaspoons your sweetener
    of choice, plus extra to taste
1 tablespoon apple cider vinegar, plus extra to taste
1 garlic clove, crushed

Combine all the ingredients in a bowl and stir well. Taste and adjust
the tamari, vinegar and stevia as desired.

---

4 RANCH DRESSING

▲ WF ▲ GF ▲ SF ▲ NF

MAKES 250 ML (9 FL OZ/1 CUP)

260 g (9¼ oz/1 cup) Greek-style full-fat yoghurt
1 teaspoon apple cider vinegar
1 teaspoon lemon juice
½ teaspoon sugar-free dijon mustard
1 garlic clove, crushed
½ teaspoon Celtic sea salt
½ teaspoon freshly cracked black pepper
2 teaspoons chopped flat-leaf (Italian) parsley
2 tablespoons grated parmesan

Combine all the ingredients and chill before serving.

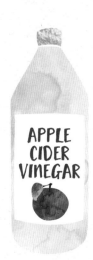

APPLE
CIDER
VINEGAR

5 HUMMUS THE HERO

▲ WF   ▲ DF   ▲ GF   ▲ SF   ▲ VG   ▲ NF

MAKES ABOUT 220 G (7 ¾ OZ/1 CUP)

400 g (14 oz) tin chickpeas, rinsed and drained
60 ml (2 fl oz/¼ cup) extra virgin olive oil
1 teaspoon grated lemon zest
1 tablespoon lemon juice
1 teaspoon ground cumin

Whizz all the ingredients together in a food processor until smooth and creamy. Serve with vegies, 4 pm Pick-up bicks (page 78), or rice or gluten-free crackers.

 SUPERCHARGED TIP This dip can be stored in an airtight container in the fridge for up to 4 days.

---

6 GUACAMOLE

▲ WF   ▲ DF   ▲ GF   ▲ SF   ▲ VG   ▲ NF

MAKES ABOUT 250 ML (9 FL OZ/1 CUP)

2 ripe avocados, seeded and peeled
juice of 1 lime
1 small onion, chopped
1 garlic clove, crushed
1 tomato, diced
Celtic sea salt and freshly cracked black pepper, to taste

Mash the avocado with the lime juice. Add the remaining ingredients and stir to combine.

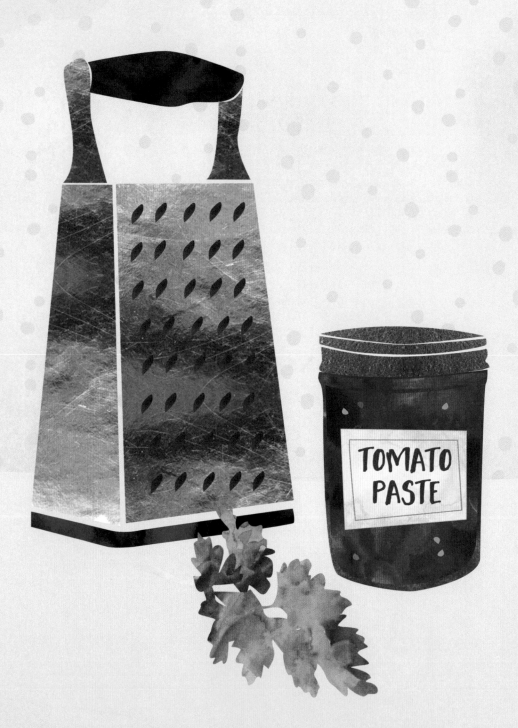

HEALTHY MEALS

Turn the page for a selection of delicious meals
that will satisfy fussy eaters and
rumbling tummies.

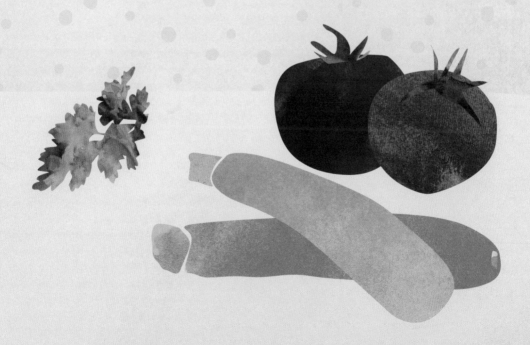

VEGIE-PACKED LAMB MEATBALLS

▲ WF　▲ DF　▲ GF　▲ SF　▲ NF

SERVES 3

> 1 tablespoon extra virgin coconut oil, plus extra as needed
> 1 onion, finely chopped
> 2 garlic cloves, crushed
> 1 carrot, finely grated
> 2 tablespoons tomato paste (concentrated purée)
> 1 zucchini (courgette)
> 2 tablespoons flat-leaf (Italian) parsley
> 500 g (1 lb 2 oz) minced (ground) lamb
> Celtic sea salt, to taste
> dulse flakes, to taste (optional)

Heat the coconut oil in a frying pan over medium heat. Add the onion and garlic, and cook for 3–4 minutes or until translucent. Add the carrot and tomato paste, and cook for 5 minutes. Remove from the heat and set aside to cool. Keep the oily pan ready to use again.

Finely chop the zucchini and parsley in a food processor. Transfer to a sieve and squeeze out any excess moisture, then set aside in a large bowl. Add the lamb, onion mix, salt and dulse flakes (if using), and mix well.

Use your hands to form walnut-sized balls. Return the frying pan to medium heat and cook the meatballs for 10 minutes, adding a little more oil if necessary, until browned on all sides and cooked through.

 SUPERCHARGED TIP Make these meatballs ahead of time and freeze them to cut down meal-prep time on a busy night.

HEALTH TIP Fussy eaters won't know what's hit them when their scrummy favourites are full of hidden vegetables.

CRUNCHY CHICKEN DRUMMERS

▲ WF ▲ GF ▲ SF ▲ NF

SERVES 4

2 tablespoons melted butter
90 g (3¼ oz) brown rice crackers
8 chicken drumsticks, skin removed if preferred
1 large egg, lightly beaten

Preheat the oven to 200°C (400°F). Line a roasting tin with foil and brush with the melted butter.

Place the brown rice crackers in a zip-lock bag. Close the bag and crush the contents to fine crumbs with a rolling pin. Dip one or two drumsticks at a time in the egg, then add to the zip-lock bag and shake to coat the chicken evenly.

Transfer to the prepared roasting tin and bake for 30–35 minutes or until the chicken is cooked through and the coating is browned and crispy.

 SUPERCHARGED TIP When cooking this recipe, always make extra! They're a great addition to the lunchbox when cold. Just ensure they'll stay cold until lunchtime.

TOMATO TUBS WITH TUNA

WF DF GF SF NF

MAKES 4

4 tomatoes
185 g (6$\frac{1}{2}$ oz/1 cup) cooked brown rice (from about
   80 g/2$\frac{3}{4}$ oz uncooked rice), or 220 g (7 oz/1 cup)
   cooked quinoa (from about 55 g/2 oz uncooked quinoa)
400 g (14 oz) tin tuna, drained
Celtic sea salt and freshly cracked black pepper, to taste
handful of basil leaves, chopped

Slice a thin piece off the top of each tomato and set aside. Hollow out the tomatoes (setting aside the flesh for another use, such as a pasta sauce). Combine the rice and tuna in a bowl, season with salt and pepper, then spoon into the tomatoes.

Top with the basil, and the reserved tomato lid, then serve. (Alternatively, arrange the tomatoes in a small roasting tin or baking dish – so that they hold each other up and don't fall over during cooking – and bake in a 160°C/315°F oven for 25–30 minutes or until the tomatoes are tender.)

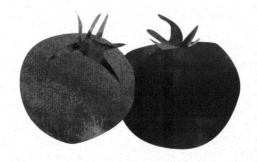

VEGIE NOUGHTS AND CROSSES

▲ SF ▲ NF

SERVES 2

2 slices brown rice or buckwheat bread
1 slice sourdough bread
2 teaspoons Hummus the hero (page 101)
2 teaspoons Cucumber and yoghurt dip (page 99)
1 celery stalk
4 thin slices carrot

Cut five 4 cm (1½ inch) squares from the brown rice bread and four 4 cm
(1½ inch) squares from the sourdough and set aside. Spread the sourdough
squares with hummus and the brown rice bread squares with yoghurt dip.

On a large platter or tray, arrange the bread squares to form a checkerboard
pattern with the brown rice bread in the corners and centre. Cut ten 5 cm
(2 inch) long thin pieces from the celery stalk to make crosses and place on
the brown rice squares, then place the carrot slices on the sourdough
squares to make noughts.

 SUPERCHARGED TIP Use a slice of Seeded loaf (page 125)
in place of the sourdough loaf to boost the nutritional intake
and cater for children who can't eat gluten.

ZUCCHINI SLICE

▲ WF   ▲ GF   ▲ SF   ▲ NF

SERVES 3–4

butter, for greasing
1 onion, diced
4 slices bacon, diced
3 zucchini (courgettes), grated
2 carrots, grated
100 g (3½ oz/1 cup) grated cheddar cheese
100 g (3½ oz/²/₃ cup) gluten-free self-raising flour
1 teaspoon gluten-free baking powder
5 eggs, lightly beaten

Preheat the oven to 180°C (350°F) and grease a 20 cm (8 inch) round quiche or pie dish.

Combine all the ingredients in a large bowl and mix with a wooden spoon. Pour into the prepared quiche or pie dish. Bake for 45–50 minutes or until set.

HEALTH TIP Zucchini is high in fibre and can therefore help maintain healthy bowel function.

MINI SALMON FRITTATAS

▲ WF ▲ GF ▲ SF ▲ NF

MAKES 12

butter, for greasing
60 g (2¼ oz/ ½ cup) goat's cheese or grated cheddar
2 spring onions (scallions), finely chopped
4 eggs, lightly beaten
30 g (1 oz/ ½ cup) broccoli florets, lightly steamed
100 g (3½ oz) tin salmon, drained
Celtic sea salt and freshly cracked black pepper, to taste
dulse flakes, to taste (optional)

Preheat the oven to 190°C (375°F) and grease a 12 x 80 ml (2½ fl oz/ ⅓ cup)
hole muffin tin with the butter.

Combine all the ingredients in a bowl and mix with a wooden spoon. Divide
the salmon mixture among the muffin holes. Bake for 15 minutes or until firm
and golden.

 SUPERCHARGED TIP Freeze these frittatas and thaw one
or two for a quick and healthy after-school snack.

HEALTH TIP Full of good fats, salmon should be included in your diet
at least twice a week. It has a powerful anti-inflammatory effect and is full
of antioxidants such as vitamins B, D and E, which help boost immunity.

LAMB SAUSAGE AND BASIL EGG MUFFINS

△ DF ▲ SF ▲ NF

SERVES 12

coconut oil, for greasing
10 eggs, lightly beaten
15 g (¹/₂ oz/ ¹/₄ cup) chopped basil
Celtic sea salt and freshly cracked black pepper, to taste
500 g (1 lb 2 oz) lamb sausages, cooked, cooled and chopped
  into bite-sized pieces

Preheat the oven to 180°C (350°F) and grease a 12 x 80 ml (2¹/₂ fl oz/ ¹/₃ cup) hole muffin tin.

Combine the eggs with the basil in a bowl and season with salt and pepper. Divide the sausage evenly between the muffin holes. Pour the egg mixture over the top and bake for 15–20 minutes or until set.

Remove from the oven and allow to cool for about 5 minutes before loosening with a knife. Serve warm or cold.

 SUPERCHARGED TIP These muffins will keep in an airtight container in the fridge for up to 3 days.

HEALTH TIP This high-energy meal will keep the kids active and alert.

ZUCCHINI FRITTERS

▲ WF   ▲ DF   ▲ GF   ▲ SF

MAKES 10

2 zucchini (courgettes), grated
1 teaspoon Celtic sea salt, plus extra to taste
2 spring onions (scallions), cut in half lengthways and thinly sliced
1 large egg, lightly beaten
freshly cracked black pepper, to taste
50 g (1³/₄ oz/ ¹/₂ cup) almond meal
¹/₂ teaspoon gluten-free baking powder
coconut oil, for shallow-frying

Preheat the oven to 200°C (400°F).

Place the zucchini in a sieve over a bowl. Add the salt and set aside for 20 minutes. Squeeze the zucchini to remove all of the excess moisture, then transfer to a bowl. Add the spring onion, egg, pepper, almond meal and baking powder, and stir well.

Heat the oil in a frying pan over medium-high heat and drop 2 tablespoons of the mixture into the pan. Flatten with the back of a spatula and cook for 4 minutes until golden, then turn and cook for 4 minutes on the other side. Repeat with the remaining mixture.

Serve two fritters per child.

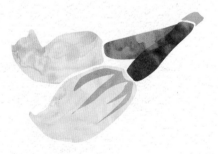

HAM AND CHEESE PIZZA

▲ WF ▲ GF ▲ SF

MAKES 2

PIZZA BASES
150 g (5½ oz/ 1½ cups) almond meal, plus extra as needed
2 eggs, lightly beaten
2 tablespoons extra virgin olive oil
2 tablespoons nutritional yeast flakes
½ teaspoon dried oregano
½ teaspoon dried basil
2 garlic cloves, crushed
¼ teaspoon Celtic sea salt
1 teaspoon apple cider vinegar

TOPPING
2 tablespoons tomato paste (concentrated purée)
105 g (3¾ oz/ ½ cup) oven-roasted tomatoes (optional)
65 g (2¼ oz/ ⅔ cup) grated cheddar cheese or goat's cheese
80 g (2¾ oz/ ½ cup) chopped ham
dulse flakes, for sprinkling (optional)

Preheat the oven to 220°C (425°F) and lightly grease two small pizza pans.

To prepare the pizza bases, combine all the ingredients in a large mixing bowl to form a loose dough. If it feels wet, add a little more almond meal. Dust the bench with almond meal and knead the dough with your hands until smooth. Shape into a ball. Cut the dough in half and roll each portion out into a thin circle about 15 cm (6 inch) in diameter, working from the inside out in a clockwise motion. Add more almond meal if it becomes too sticky. Place the bases on the prepared pizza pans and bake for 10 minutes.

Remove the bases from the oven and spread with tomato paste, leaving a 1 cm (½ inch) border. Scatter over the tomatoes, if using, and the cheese and ham, and sprinkle with dulse flakes, if using. Return the pizzas to the oven for 7-10 minutes, or until crispy.

 SUPERCHARGED TIP You can freeze the bases before rolling and defrost when required.

CHICKEN BALLS WITH SWEET POTATO MASH

▲ WF   ▲ GF   ▲ SF   ▲ NF

SERVES 4

2 large sweet potatoes
185 g (6½ oz/1 cup) cooked brown rice
½ onion, finely diced
½ red capsicum (pepper), seeded and puréed in a blender
handful of coriander (cilantro), chopped
1 garlic clove, crushed
500 g (1 lb 2 oz) minced (ground) chicken
coconut oil, for shallow-frying
2 tablespoons butter
2 teaspoons ground cinnamon

Preheat the oven to 200°C (400°F).

Wash and dry the sweet potatoes, then wrap individually in foil.
Bake them on a baking tray for 90 minutes or until soft. Set aside.

Combine the rice, onion, capsicum, coriander and garlic in a bowl and
stir well. Stir in the chicken. Roll the mixture into walnut-sized balls.

Heat a little coconut oil in a frying pan over medium heat. Add the
meatballs and cook for 10 minutes, turning regularly to cook all over.

Scoop the flesh out of the sweet potatoes and transfer to a bowl.
Add the butter and cinnamon, and mash until smooth.

Serve the meatballs on a bed of sweet potato mash.

FRESH TUNA PASTA WITH ZUCCHINI

▲ WF ▲ DF ▲ GF ▲ SF ▲ NF

SERVES 4

2 x 150–200 g (5½–7 oz) fresh tuna fillets
2 tablespoons extra virgin olive oil, plus extra for drizzling
2 garlic cloves, crushed
1 onion, finely sliced
3 zucchini (courgettes), cut in half lengthways then sliced
360 g (12¾ oz/4 cups) gluten-free penne pasta
Celtic sea salt and freshly cracked black pepper, to taste
chopped flat-leaf (Italian) parsley, to serve

Wash the tuna and pat dry with paper towel. Heat half the olive oil
in a frying pan over medium heat. Add the tuna and sear for 2 minutes
on each side. Set aside.

Heat the remaining olive oil in the same pan, then add the garlic and onion,
and cook for 3–4 minutes or until translucent. Add the zucchini and cook,
stirring frequently, for 10 minutes or until the zucchini is cooked through.

Meanwhile, cook the pasta until al dente in plenty of boiling salted water
according to the packet instructions. Drain, reserving a few tablespoons
of the cooking water.

Add the pasta to the pan with the zucchini, stir well and let it cook with
the zucchini for 1 minute. Flake the tuna and add to the pan. Mix well,
adding some reserved pasta-cooking water, if necessary.

Season and serve with parsley and a drizzle of olive oil.

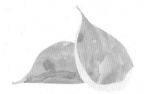

CAULIFLOWER MAC AND CHEESE

⚠ WF ⚠ GF ⚠ SF ⚠ NF

SERVES 4

1 tablespoon butter, plus extra for greasing
1 teaspoon Celtic sea salt
1 large cauliflower, cut into small florets
250 ml (9 fl oz/1 cup) thick (double/heavy) cream
90 g (3¼ oz/¾ cup) goat's cheese
1 teaspoon sugar-free dijon mustard
150 g (5½ oz/1½ cups) grated cheddar cheese
Celtic sea salt and freshly cracked black pepper, to taste
90 g (3¼ oz/1 cup) cooked buckwheat or gluten-free pasta
15 g (½ oz/½ cup) brown rice puffs

Preheat the oven to 190°C (375°F) and grease a baking dish.

Bring a large saucepan of water to the boil and add the salt. Add the cauliflower and cook for 10 minutes or until al dente. Drain well, then transfer to the prepared baking dish and set aside.

Bring the butter and cream to a simmer in a small saucepan, then whisk in the goat's cheese and mustard until smooth. Stir in 100 g (3½ oz/1 cup) of the cheddar, and whisk for 1–2 minutes or until it just melts.

Pour the sauce over the cauliflower, add the cooked pasta and stir to combine. Top with the remaining cheddar and the brown rice puffs, then bake for 15 minutes or until browned and bubbly.

 SUPERCHARGED TIP Just a few switches make this old favourite a meal every kid will enjoy.

HEALTH TIP Cauliflower is full of antioxidants and vitamin C, and contains omega-3 fatty acids. Eat up!

NEAPOLITAN MEATBALL PASTA

△ WF △ DF △ GF △ NF
SERVES 4

360 g (12³/₄ oz/4 cups) gluten-free spiral pasta
Celtic sea salt, to taste
basil leaves, torn, plus extra to serve

MEATBALLS
400 g (14 oz) minced (ground) lamb
1 egg, lightly beaten
2 garlic cloves, crushed
handful of basil, finely chopped
pinch of ground nutmeg
pinch of ground cinnamon
1 teaspoon grated lemon zest
Celtic sea salt and freshly cracked black pepper, to taste
coconut flour, for dusting
extra virgin olive oil, for shallow-frying

SAUCE
1 tablespoon extra virgin olive oil
2 garlic cloves, crushed
1 small onion, finely chopped
520 g (1 lb 2 oz/2 cups) tomato passata (puréed tomatoes)
200 g (7 oz/1 cup) chopped roma (plum) tomatoes
1 tablespoon balsamic vinegar
Celtic sea salt, to taste
1 tablespoon rice malt syrup or a few drops stevia (optional)

To prepare the meatballs, combine all the ingredients except the flour and olive oil in a large bowl. Work with your hands to obtain a smooth mixture. If the mixture is too sloppy, add a little coconut flour. Set aside.

To prepare the sauce, heat the olive oil in a large saucepan over medium heat. Add the garlic and onion, and cook for 4 minutes or until softened. Add the passata, tomatoes, balsamic vinegar, salt and rice malt syrup or stevia, if using, and cook for 15 minutes or until the sauce has thickened.

With wet hands, form small balls of the meat mixture. Roll them in coconut flour to cover them evenly. Heat a little olive oil in a large frying pan over medium heat and cook the meatballs for about 10 minutes or until they're browned all over.

Add the meatballs to the sauce and cook gently for 12–15 minutes or until cooked through.

While the sauce and meatballs are cooking, cook the pasta in plenty of boiling salted water according to the packet instructions. Drain, then add to the sauce and meatballs.

Stir through the basil and simmer for 1 minute. Serve topped with extra torn basil.

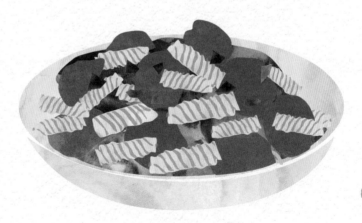

LENTIL POT PIES

▲ WF ▲ GF ▲ SF ▲ NF
SERVES 4

1 tablespoon extra virgin olive oil
1 onion, finely chopped
135 g (4¾ oz/1½ cups) chopped mushrooms
1 zucchini (courgette), finely diced
3 garlic cloves, crushed
pinch of dried oregano
1–2 teaspoons dried thyme
1 carrot, diced
170 g (6 oz/¾ cup) brown lentils, rinsed
750 ml (26 fl oz/3 cups) vegetable stock
1 tablespoon wheat-free tamari
75 g (2½ oz/½ cup) frozen or fresh peas

CAULIFLOWER MASH
1 cauliflower, cut into florets
1 tablespoon butter (or light olive oil or almond milk for vegans)
1 tablespoon nutritional yeast flakes
pinch of Celtic sea salt
freshly cracked black pepper, to taste

To prepare the cauliflower mash, steam the cauliflower for 10 minutes or until tender – it should be soft but not falling apart. Transfer to a blender or food processor with the butter, yeast flakes, salt and pepper. Blend until smooth then set aside.

Preheat the oven to 200°C (400°F). Heat the olive oil in a medium saucepan over medium-high heat. Add the onion and cook for 3–4 minutes or until translucent. Add the mushroom, zucchini, garlic, oregano and thyme, and cook for 5 minutes. Add the carrot, lentils and stock. Cover and bring to the boil, then reduce the heat and simmer, uncovered, for 20 minutes or until the stock has mostly cooked away, then stir in the tamari and peas. Divide the mixture between four individual pie dishes. Spoon the cauliflower mash over the top, and decorate by scraping a fork across the surface. Bake for 20 minutes or until the top is golden.

ROCKIN' FRIED RICE

WF ⬛ DF ⬛ GF ⬛ SF ⬛ NF

SERVES 4–5

1 tablespoon extra virgin coconut oil
2 rashers bacon, finely diced
2 French shallots (eschalots), finely diced
100 g (3½ oz/⅔ cup) frozen or fresh peas
80 g (2¾ oz/¾ cup) green beans, cut into 2 cm (¾ inch) lengths
1 carrot, finely diced
925 g (2 lb 1 oz/5 cups) cooked brown rice
  (from about 400 g/14 oz/2 cups uncooked rice)
2 tablespoons wheat-free tamari
2 eggs, lightly beaten

Heat the coconut oil in a large frying pan over medium heat until sizzling. Add the bacon, shallot, peas, beans and carrot, and cook, stirring frequently, for 3–4 minutes or until lightly cooked. Add the rice and cook for 5 minutes, stirring once a minute. Stir through the tamari and cook for another 2 minutes.

Move the rice mixture over to one side of the pan and pour in the egg. Let it cook for 30 seconds, scrambling it with a fork, then mix it through the rice and serve straight away.

BREAD AND WRAP BASICS

There's nothing quite as rewarding as making your own bread, and it's great for your kids' health, too.

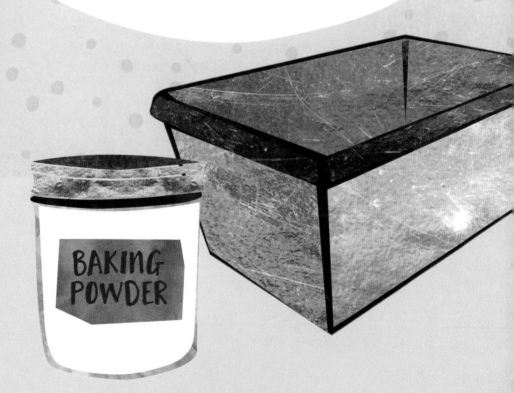

EVERYDAY GLUTEN-FREE LOAF

▲ WF   ▲ DF   ▲ GF

MAKES 1 LOAF, 21 CM X 9 CM (8¼ INCHES X 3½ INCHES)

coconut oil, for greasing
150 g (5½ oz/1½ cups) almond meal
95 g (3¼ oz/¾ cup) tapioca flour (arrowroot)
25 g (1 oz/¼ cup) flaxseed meal
½ teaspoon stevia powder
pinch of Celtic sea salt
½ teaspoon gluten-free baking powder
1 teaspoon bicarbonate of soda (baking soda)
4 eggs
1 teaspoon rice malt syrup
1 teaspoon apple cider vinegar

Preheat the oven to 175°C (345°F) and grease a 21 cm x 9 cm (8¼ inch x 3½ inch) loaf (bar) tin.

Combine the almond meal, tapioca flour, flaxseed meal, stevia, salt, baking powder and bicarbonate of soda in a large bowl. In another bowl, whisk the eggs well, then stir through the rice malt syrup and apple cider vinegar. Add the egg mixture to the dry ingredients and mix well.

Pour the batter into the prepared tin and bake for 30–35 minutes or until a skewer inserted in the centre comes out clean. Cool in the tin.

 SUPERCHARGED TIP Organic golden flaxseed meal is the product left after pressing flaxseeds to get flaxseed oil. It still contains 12 per cent fat, half of which is the omega-3 essential fatty acid alpha-linolenic acid (ALA).

COCONUT PANCAKES

▲ WF ▲ GF ▲ SF ▲ NF*

MAKES 4

2 egg whites, lightly beaten
2 tablespoons coconut flour
⅛ teaspoon bicarbonate of soda (baking soda)
⅛ teaspoon gluten-free baking powder
pinch of Celtic sea salt
125 ml (4 fl oz/½ cup) almond milk, or rice milk for nut-free*
1 tablespoon butter

Combine all the ingredients except the butter in a bowl until smooth.

Heat the butter in a heavy-based 20 cm (8 inch) frying pan over medium heat. Pour a quarter of the mixture into the pan. When it starts to bubble, carefully flip the pancake over and cook for 1 minute or until cooked through. Repeat with the remaining mixture.

Allow to cool then enjoy with your favourite toppings.

GLUTEN-FREE PITTA POCKET

▲ WF ▲ DF ▲ GF ▲ SF

MAKES 4

Stuff these with your child's favourite fillings.

1 egg
60 ml (2 fl oz/¼ cup) water
1 tablespoon almond milk or rice milk
1 tablespoon extra virgin olive oil
1 tablespoon coconut flour
1 tablespoon flaxseed meal
25 g (1 oz/¼ cup) blanched almond meal
⅛ teaspoon bicarbonate of soda (baking soda)
pinch of Celtic sea salt
1 tablespoon finely chopped herbs of your choice (optional)

Preheat the oven to 180°C (350°F). Draw two circles of about 12 cm (4½ inch) diameter on a sheet of baking paper and place on a baking tray with the side you drew on facing down.

Whisk the egg, water, milk and olive oil together in a bowl. Add the remaining ingredients and stir well.

Pour the mixture onto the baking paper in the centre of each circle and spread evenly with a palette knife to fill the circle you drew. Bake for 20 minutes or until golden and crispy around the edges.

Cool, then cut in half with a sharp knife so that a pocket is created.

SEEDED LOAF

▲ WF　▲ GF　▲ SF　▲ NF

MAKES 1 LOAF, 21 CM X 9 CM (8¼ INCHES X 3½ INCHES)

> 330 g (11½ oz/2⅓ cups) gluten-free self-raising flour,
>   plus extra for dusting
> 185 g (6½ oz/1¼ cups) mixed seeds
> ¼ teaspoon Celtic sea salt
> ¼ teaspoon stevia powder
> 4 eggs
> 1 teaspoon apple cider vinegar
> 60 g (2¼ oz) butter, melted, plus extra for greasing
> 60 ml (2 fl oz/¼ cup) additive-free coconut milk
> 125 ml (4 fl oz/½ cup) water

Preheat the oven to 175°C (345°F). Grease and flour a 21 cm x 9 cm (8¼ inch x 3½ inch) loaf (bar) tin.

Combine the flour, seeds, salt and stevia in a large bowl. In a separate bowl, beat the eggs with an electric mixer for 2 minutes until pale and fluffy. Add the vinegar, butter, coconut milk and water, and stir to combine. Add the egg mixture to the dry ingredients and mix well.

Spoon into the prepared tin, smooth the surface with the back of a spoon and bake for 40 minutes, or until a skewer inserted into the centre of the loaf comes out clean. Turn out onto a wire rack to cool.

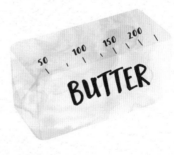

CREPE WRAPS

△ WF △ GF ▲ SF △ NF

MAKES 3

This recipe for crepes is so easy – and they're versatile, too. You can use them to make delicious gluten-free wraps for lunchboxes or top them with berries and goat's cheese for breakfast for the whole family.

130 g (4$\frac{1}{2}$ oz/1 cup) tapioca flour (arrowroot)
250 ml (9 fl oz/1 cup) additive-free coconut milk
1 egg
pinch of Celtic sea salt
60 g (2$\frac{1}{4}$ oz) butter

Combine all the ingredients except the butter in a medium bowl and stir well.

Heat one-third of the butter in a frying pan over medium heat. Pour in one-third of the mixture and swirl to cover the bottom of the pan. After 2–3 minutes, carefully flip and brown on the other side. Repeat with the remaining butter and crepe mixture.

ALMOND AND ZUCCHINI BREAD

WF   DF   GF   SF

MAKES 1 LOAF, 21 CM X 9 CM (8¼ INCHES X 3½ INCHES)

270 g (9½ oz) zucchini (courgettes), grated
½ teaspoon stevia powder
65 g (2¼ oz/½ cup) buckwheat flour or your flour of choice
200 g (7 oz/2 cups) almond meal
1 teaspoon Celtic sea salt
1 teaspoon bicarbonate of soda (baking soda)
½ teaspoon gluten-free baking powder
1 teaspoon ground cinnamon
125 ml (4 fl oz/½ cup) grapeseed oil, or 125 g (4½ oz) butter,
  melted (if tolerated)
3 eggs
60 ml (2 fl oz/¼ cup) additive-free coconut milk
1 teaspoon lemon juice

Preheat the oven to 175°C (345°F) and grease a 21 cm x 9 cm (8¼ inch x 3½ inch) loaf (bar) tin. Squeeze the zucchini with paper towel to remove excess moisture.

Combine the stevia, buckwheat flour, almond meal, salt, bicarbonate of soda, baking powder and cinnamon in a bowl, and stir well. In a separate bowl, whisk together the grapeseed oil, eggs, coconut milk and lemon juice. Add the egg mixture and the zucchini to the dry ingredients and stir well to combine.

Spoon into the prepared tin and bake on the middle rack of the oven for 45 minutes or until a skewer inserted into the centre comes out clean. Turn out onto a wire rack to cool.

BANANA BREAD

▲ WF ▲ DF ▲ GF

MAKES 1 LOAF, 21 CM X 9 CM (8¼ INCHES X 3½ INCHES)

200 g (7 oz/2 cups) almond meal
70 g (2½ oz/½ cup) walnuts, finely chopped
½ teaspoon gluten-free baking powder
1 teaspoon bicarbonate of soda (baking soda)
½ teaspoon Celtic sea salt
1 teaspoon ground cinnamon
½ teaspoon ground nutmeg
1 teaspoon alcohol-free vanilla extract
8 drops liquid stevia
3 eggs
125 ml (4 fl oz/½ cup) grapeseed oil or light olive oil
60 ml (2 fl oz/¼ cup) additive-free coconut milk
3 bananas, mashed

Preheat the oven to 170°C (325°F) and grease a 21 cm x 11 cm (8¼ inch x 4¼ inch) loaf (bar) tin.

Combine the almond meal, walnuts, baking powder, bicarbonate of soda, salt, cinnamon, nutmeg, vanilla and stevia in a bowl and stir well. In another bowl, whisk together the eggs, grapeseed oil and coconut milk. Add to the dry ingredients and stir through. Add the mashed banana and stir through until just combined.

Spoon the batter into the prepared tin and bake for 30–40 minutes or until a skewer inserted into the centre of the loaf comes out clean. Cool in the tin for 10 minutes before turning out onto a wire rack to cool completely.

10 LUNCHBOX IDEAS
WITH SANDWICHES AND WRAPS

Here are some lunchbox sandwich and wrap ideas using your favourite store-bought bread options, or one of the basic breads or wraps in the previous pages.

✶ Sardine and tomato toasties on two slices of Seeded loaf (page 125)

✶ Cheesy bacon and egg scramble (page 62) in a Crepe wrap (page 126)

✶ Gluten-free pitta pocket (page 124) filled with shredded iceberg lettuce, cucumber, carrot and Ranch dressing (page 100)

✶ Sausages, grated cheese and tomato in a gluten-free wrap

✶ Lamb sandwiches on brown rice or buckwheat bread with Cucumber and yoghurt dip (page 99)

✶ Tuna and egg in a Crepe wrap (page 126) with pesto

✶ Toasted chicken breast sandwich on Seeded loaf (page 125) with Guacamole (page 101)

✶ Falafel and Hummus the hero (page 101) wrapped in a Coconut pancake (page 123)

✶ Roasted vegetables with haloumi or goat's cheese in a Gluten-free pitta pocket (page 124)

✶ Ham, cheese and cucumber sandwich on Seeded loaf (page 125)

MONDAY TO FRIDAY
LUNCHBOX MENU

See the kids' faces light up when they can plan their own lunchbox menu for the week. Skip the same old tired sandwiches and take lunch to the next level. Here's a guide for you to follow then add your own ideas.

MONDAY

✳ Superhero chocolate milk (page 50)

✳ Supercharged breakfast bar (page 60)

✳ Mini spring roll (page 86)

✳ Celery and carrots with nut butter dipping sauce (page 80)

✳ Apple

✳ Water

TUESDAY

✳ Very berry shake (page 52)

✳ Chia coconut pikelet (page 65) with banana

✳ Toasted chicken breast sandwich on Seeded loaf (page 125) with Guacamole (page 101)

✳ Orange segments

✳ Water

WEDNESDAY

* Sparkling water with lemon

* French toast (page 59)

* Chicken nuggets (page 85) with Sweet and sour potato fries with apple cider vinegar (page 75)

* Berries with full-fat plain yoghurt

* Water

THURSDAY

* Supercharged green slushie (page 52)

* Orange and cranberry muffin (page 82)

* Ham, cheese and cucumber sandwich on Seeded loaf (page 125)

* Pirate muesli bar (page 83)

* Water

FRIDAY

* Pink lemonade (page 50)

* Cacao bomb crackle (page 76)

* Lentil pot pies (page 118) with Apple slaw (page 94)

* Yoghurt berry crunch pot (page 138)

* Water

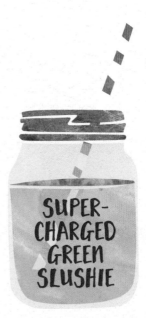

SUPER-CHARGED GREEN SLUSHIE

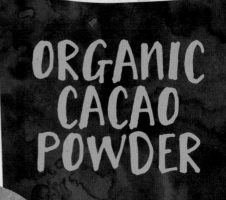
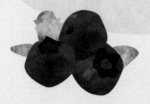

ORGANIC
CACAO
POWDER

DESSERTS

Nutritious, tasty and simple to prepare,
these crave-worthy and kid-friendly desserts knock
the socks off sugar-filled creations.

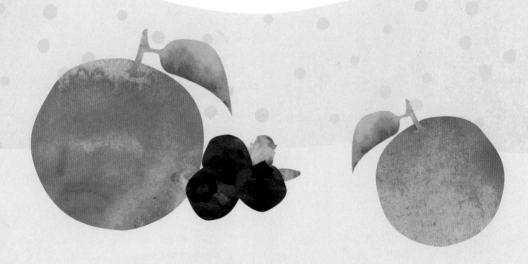

BANANA ICE CREAM

▲ WF　▲ DF　▲ GF　▲ VG

SERVES 2–3

2 bananas, peeled, frozen and cut into chunks
1 tablespoon cacao powder
6 drops liquid stevia or 2 teaspoons your sweetener of choice
1 tablespoon almond butter

Whizz all the ingredients in a food processor until creamy, scraping the sides as necessary. Serve immediately.

BLUEBERRY RICE CRISPY BARS

▲ WF　▲ DF　▲ GF　▲ VG

MAKES 20

225 g (8 oz/1$\frac{1}{2}$ cups) nuts or seeds of your choice
160 g (5$\frac{1}{2}$ oz/1 cup) dried blueberries
190 g (6$\frac{3}{4}$ oz/$\frac{3}{4}$ cup) nut butter
270 g (9$\frac{1}{2}$ oz/$\frac{3}{4}$ cup) rice malt syrup
1 teaspoon alcohol-free vanilla extract
100 g (3$\frac{1}{2}$ oz/4 cups) brown rice puffs
pinch of Celtic sea salt

Line a 20 cm (8 inch) square tin with baking paper.

Process the nuts or seeds and blueberries in a food processor until roughly ground. Combine the nut butter, rice malt syrup and vanilla in a medium saucepan over low heat, and stir until combined. Remove from the heat, then add the blueberry mix and brown rice puffs. Stir to coat. Add the salt.

Spoon into the prepared tin, pressing it down with your hands and levelling it with a spatula. Refrigerate until set, then cut into 20 bars of 2 cm x 10 cm ($\frac{3}{4}$ inches x 4 inches) or 4 cm x 5 cm (1$\frac{1}{2}$ inches x 2 inches). Refrigerate.

FRUITY SAILING BOATS

△ WF △ DF △ GF △ VG △ NF

SERVES 1–2

To make these you'll need skewers and a piece of cardboard (card) about 10 cm (4 inches) square. You can vary the fruit as you like.

> 1 apple
> 1 banana, sliced
> 90 g (3¼ oz/½ cup) grapes
> 70 g (2½ oz/½ cup) mixed berries

Slice the top off the apple and carefully scoop out the flesh using a knife and spoon. Dice the apple flesh, add to a bowl with the other fruit and mix through. Spoon into the apple shell.

Fold the cardboard in half diagonally and cut it into a triangle. Cut two slits in the middle of the triangle and place a skewer through the slits, pointy end towards the bottom of the 'sail'. Place the sail in the apple 'boat' and serve immediately.

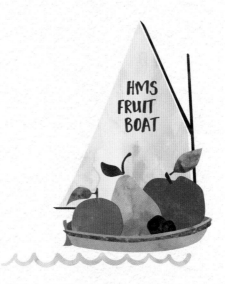

CHOCOLATE CAKE

▲ WF ▲ GF ▲ NF

MAKES 1 CAKE, 21 CM X 9 CM (8¼ INCHES X 3½ INCHES)

Slice this one up for the lunchbox.

90 g (3¼ oz/¾ cup) coconut flour
55 g (2 oz/½ cup) cacao powder
1 teaspoon Celtic sea salt
1 teaspoon gluten-free baking powder
6 eggs
250 g (9 oz) butter, melted
540 g (1 lb 3 oz/1½ cups) rice malt syrup
1 teaspoon alcohol-free vanilla extract

Preheat the oven to 175°C (345°F) and line a 21 cm x 9 cm (8¼ inch x 3½ inch) loaf (bar) tin with baking paper.

Combine the flour, cacao, salt and baking powder in a bowl. In a separate large bowl, whisk together the eggs, butter, rice malt syrup and vanilla. Add the dry ingredients to the egg mixture and mix well.

Pour the batter into the prepared tin and bake for 40 minutes or until a skewer inserted into the centre comes out clean. Turn out onto a wire rack to cool.

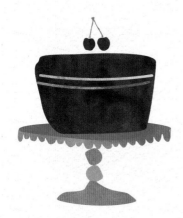

ORANGE AND POPPY SEED CAKE

▲ WF ◢ DF ▲ GF

MAKES 1 CAKE, 21 CM X 9 CM (8¼ INCHES X 3½ INCHES)

> 2 oranges
> 6 eggs
> 285 g (10 oz/1½ cups) xylitol
> 150 g (5½ oz/1½ cups) almond meal
> 3 teaspoons gluten-free baking powder
> 2 tablespoons poppy seeds

Cut off and discard the tops of the oranges and score the cut surface with a cross about 3 cm (1¼ inches) deep. Place the oranges in a saucepan of boiling water and boil for 45 minutes. Drain and set aside to cool.

Preheat the oven to 160°C (315°F) and line a 21 cm x 9 cm (8¼ inch x 3½ inch) loaf (bar) tin with baking paper.

Whizz the oranges in a food processor until smooth.

In a large mixing bowl, whisk the eggs with the xylitol until light and fluffy. Add the almond meal and baking powder, and stir to combine. Add the orange purée and poppy seeds, and stir well.

Spoon the mixture into the prepared tin and bake for 40 minutes. Cool in the tin for 10 minutes, then turn out onto a wire rack to cool completely.

YOGHURT BERRY CRUNCH POT

▲ WF ▲ GF ▲ NF

SERVES 2-3

200 g (7 oz/1 cup) quinoa, rinsed and drained
55 g (2 oz/⅓ cup) sunflower seeds
½ teaspoon ground cinnamon
½ teaspoon alcohol-free vanilla extract
1 tablespoon rice malt syrup
260 g (9¼ oz/1 cup) plain full-fat yoghurt
70 g (2½ oz/½ cup) fresh mixed berries
2 tablespoons coconut flakes
1 tablespoon chia seeds

Preheat the oven to 190°C (375°F) and line a baking tray with baking paper.

Combine the quinoa, sunflower seeds, cinnamon, vanilla and rice malt syrup in a bowl and mix well.

Spread the mixture in a thin layer on the prepared tray and bake for 10 minutes or until crisp but not burnt. Set aside to cool then break into little pieces.

Spoon a layer of yoghurt into each glass, alternating it with layers of crunch, then top with the berries and coconut flakes. Sprinkle with chia seeds and serve.

FRUIT SCONES

▲ WF ▲ DF* ▲ GF

MAKES 12

250 g (9 oz/2½ cups) almond meal
60 g (2¼ oz/½ cup) coconut flour
95 g (3¼ oz/½ cup) mixed dried fruit, roughly chopped
½ teaspoon Celtic sea salt
pinch of ground cinnamon
¾ teaspoon bicarbonate of soda (baking soda)
½ teaspoon vanilla powder
2 large eggs
55 g (2 oz) extra virgin coconut oil, melted
2 tablespoons rice malt syrup
plain full-fat yoghurt, to serve (omit for dairy-free*)

Preheat the oven to 180°C (350°F) and line a baking tray with baking paper.

Combine the almond meal, coconut flour, dried fruit, salt, cinnamon, bicarbonate of soda and vanilla in a large bowl and mix well. In a separate bowl, whisk together the eggs, coconut oil and rice malt syrup. Add the dry ingredients to the egg mixture and mix well, then roll spoonfuls of batter into balls and place on the prepared tray. Bake for 20 minutes or until golden.

Cool on a wire rack, then slice the scones through the middle and fill with yoghurt.

'STRAYA DAY LAMINGTONS

▲ WF　▲ DF　▲ GF

MAKES 12

6 large eggs
2 tablespoons rice malt syrup
1 teaspoon alcohol-free vanilla extract
55 g (2 oz) extra virgin coconut oil, melted
60 g (2¼ oz/½ cup) coconut flour
1½ teaspoon gluten-free baking powder
180 g (6¼ oz/2 cups) desiccated coconut

ICING
110 g (3¾ oz/½ cup) extra virgin coconut oil
45 g (1½ oz) coconut butter
55 g (2 oz/½ cup) cacao powder
60 ml (2 fl oz/¼ cup) almond milk
90 g (3¼ oz/¼ cup) rice malt syrup
pinch of ground cinnamon
1 teaspoon alcohol-free vanilla extract

Preheat the oven to 160°C (315°F). Grease and line a 20 cm (8 inch) square cake tin.

Using an electric mixer, beat the eggs with the rice malt syrup and vanilla until light and fluffy. Beat in the coconut oil, then gradually beat in the coconut flour and baking powder until smooth. Spoon the batter into the prepared tin and bake for 25–30 minutes or until golden brown and a skewer inserted into the centre comes out clean. Remove from the tin and cool on a wire rack.

To make the icing, stir all the ingredients together in a bowl until smooth. Spread out the desiccated coconut on a plate. When the cake is cool, slice into squares and dip each square into the icing, coating well. Roll in the coconut, ensuring all sides are covered. Refrigerate to set the icing.

The lamingtons will keep in an airtight container in the fridge for 3 days.

COCONUT BARS

▲ WF ▲ DF ▲ GF ▲ NF*

MAKES 10

3 eggs
185 ml (6 fl oz/ ¾ cup) additive-free coconut milk
60 g (2¼ oz) coconut butter
120 g (4¼ oz/ ⅓ cup) rice malt syrup
1 teaspoon alcohol-free vanilla extract
⅛ teaspoon stevia
50 g (1¾ oz/ ½ cup) almond meal, or flaxseed meal for nut-free*
1 tablespoon coconut flour
85 g (3 oz/1½ cups) coconut flakes
pinch of Celtic sea salt

Preheat the oven to 175°C (345°F) and grease a 20 cm (8 inch) square cake tin.

Pulse the eggs, coconut milk and butter, rice malt syrup, vanilla and stevia in a food processor to combine. Transfer to a bowl and stir in the remaining ingredients. Spoon the mixture into the prepared cake tin and bake for 20–25 minutes or until firm.

Cool in the tin, then cut into bars and refrigerate to harden.

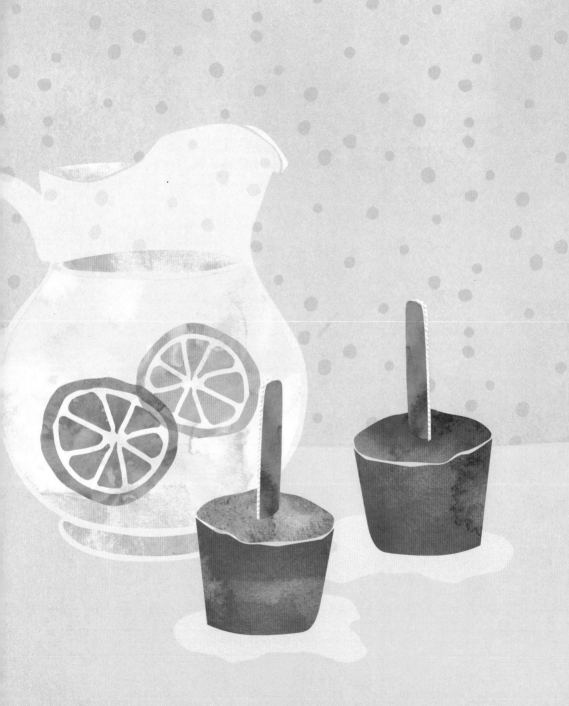

PUSH-UPS AND ICY POLES

No kid can resist a frozen treat! Make your own and you'll know they're healthy.

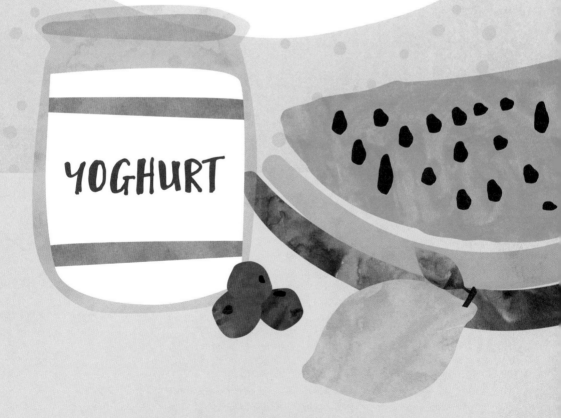

CHOCOLATE POPSICLES

▲ WF ▲ DF ▲ GF ▲ VG

MAKES 4

2 bananas
65 g (2¼ oz/¼ cup) nut butter
60 ml (2 fl oz/¼ cup) additive-free coconut milk or coconut water
2 tablespoons cacao powder
1 teaspoon alcohol-free vanilla extract
¼ teaspoon stevia powder or your sweetener of choice
4 iceblock (popsicle/ice lolly) moulds and sticks

Whizz all the ingredients in a food processor to combine.

Pour into the iceblock moulds and add the sticks, then freeze until set.

LEMONADE PUSH-UPS

▲ WF ▲ DF ▲ GF ▲ SF ▲ VG ▲ NF

MAKES 4

2 tablespoons lemon juice
500 ml (17 fl oz/2 cups) coconut water
½ teaspoon stevia powder
4 push-up moulds

Combine the lemon juice, coconut water and stevia in a jug and stir well.

Pour into the push-up moulds and freeze until set.

WATERMELON ICY POLES

⚠ WF　⚠ DF　⚠ GF　⚠ VG　⚠ NF
MAKES 4

> 300 g (10¹/₂ oz/2 cups) seeded, diced watermelon
> 1 teaspoon alcohol-free vanilla extract
> a few mint sprigs
> 4 iceblock (popsicle/ice lolly) moulds and sticks

Whizz all the ingredients in a blender until smooth.

Pour into the iceblock moulds and add the sticks, then freeze until set.

YOGHURT BERRY POPSICLES

⚠ WF　⚠ GF　⚠ NF
MAKES 4

> 250 g (9 oz/2 cups) mixed berries
> juice of 1 lime
> ¹/₂ teaspoon stevia powder or your sweetener of choice
> 390 g (13³/₄ oz/1¹/₂ cups) Greek-style full-fat yoghurt
> 170 ml (5¹/₂ fl oz/²/₃ cup) additive-free coconut milk
> 4 iceblock (popsicle/ice lolly) moulds and sticks

Purée the berries, lime juice and stevia in a blender or food processor.

Combine the yoghurt and coconut milk in a bowl. Add the berry purée and swirl through.

Pour into the iceblock moulds and add the sticks, then freeze until set.

NOTES

ALTERNATIVE SWEETENERS

p. 20   In a 2004 study, researchers also found . . .: T. Tapiainen et al.,
'Effect of xylitol on growth of *Streptococcus pneumoniae* in
the presence of fructose and sorbitol', *Antimicrobial Agents
and Chemotherapy*, vol. 45, no. 1, January 2001, pp. 166–9,
ncbi.nlm.nih.gov/pmc/articles/PMC90255.

MOOD FOOD: AVOIDING THE CRAZIES

p. 34   One study found that the omega-3 . . .: A. Vinesa et al., 'The
role of 5-HT1A receptors in fish oil-mediated increased BDNF
expression in the rat hippocampus and cortex: a possible
antidepressant mechanism', *Neuropharmacology*, vol. 62, no.
1, January 2012, pp. 184–91, sciencedirect.com/science/
journal/00283908/62/1.

A GUIDE TO THE ICONS

p. 42   In Australia, New Zealand, the United Kingdom and the
United States. . .: 'Cow's milk (dairy) allergy', January 2010,
ASCIA, allergy.org.au/patients/food-allergy/cows-milk-dairy-
allergy; Act on Cow's Milk Allergy, cowsmilkallergy.co.uk/
home; and 'Milk allergy', Asthma and Allergy Foundation
of America, aafa.org/display.cfm?id=9&sub=20&cont=516

p. 43   Researchers have shown that a child ...: N. Sinn & J. Bryan,
'Effect of supplementation with polyunsaturated fatty acids
and micronutrients on learning and behavior problems
associated with child ADHD', *Journal of Developmental and
Behavioral Pediatrics*, vol. 28, no. 2, April 2007, pp. 82–91,
journals.lww.com/jrnldbp/Abstract/2007/04000/Effect_of_
Supplementation_with_Polyunsaturated.2.aspx.

INDEX

ACKNOWLEDGEMENTS

This book is dedicated to all the mums, dads, grandparents and caregivers who are interested in home cooking and choose to make healthy choices for the children they care for. It's not always easy finding time and energy to create a balanced meal, and I'm hoping that these quick and easy-to-make recipes from my own kitchen will be adored and gobbled up by your little ones. As a busy working mum myself, it was important for me to provide you with lots of options for delicious and nutritious meals while still enabling you to spend precious time hanging out with your family. The book features healthy versions of all my 'family favourite' recipes – I hope they'll become firm favourites for you, too, and be on high rotation in your house. I want to thank all of the families who took part in testing the recipes and providing me with honest feedback.

I'd like to also extend my heartfelt thanks and gratitude to all the hardworking and dedicated people who helped to bring this book into your hands. Thank you for giving me an outlet for my passions. Thanks to Murdoch Books; Diana Hill, the best publisher in the business; and Christine Farmer for always being a fantastic teacher and guide. Thanks also to my inspiring publishing team: Hugh Ford, Sarah Odgers, Virginia Birch, Nicola Young, Matt Hoy, Robert Gorman, Sue Hines and Patrizia Di Biase-Dyson. And a big thank you to Bennett McClenahan, Billie Sigala-Pattinson, Minnie Porter and Fletcher Stanton, my co-stars at the cover shoot, and their parents.

Special thanks to my friends, colleagues and mentors Louise Cornege, Kim Cotton, Juliet Potter, Howard Porter, Georgie Bridge, Marrianne Little, Rosana Lauria, Kristy Plumridge, Hilary Davis, Cindy Luken, Jessica Lowe, Pia Larsen, Kirsten Shanks, Ema Taylor, Grahame Grassby, Mike Conway and Cindy Sciberras.

All the love in the world to my family: Roxy, Arizona, Carol, Lorraine, Clive, Alex and Ben; my wonderful and creative daughter, Tamsin Holmes, who is a delight and an inspiration, especially in the kitchen; and my partner, Justin, who is a constant source of encouragement, support and love.

Happy cooking,
Lee xo

Published in 2016 by Murdoch Books, an imprint of Allen & Unwin
Reprinted 2016 (twice)

Murdoch Books Australia
83 Alexander Street
Crows Nest NSW 2065
Phone: +61 (0) 2 8425 0100
Fax: +61 (0) 2 9906 2218
murdochbooks.com.au
info@murdochbooks.com.au

Murdoch Books UK
Erico House, 6th Floor
93–99 Upper Richmond Road
Putney, London SW15 2TG
Phone: +44 (0) 20 8785 5995
murdochbooks.co.uk
info@murdochbooks.co.uk

For Corporate Orders & Custom Publishing contact
Noel Hammond, National Business Development
Manager, Murdoch Books Australia

Publisher: Diana Hill
Editorial Manager: Virginia Birch
Design Manager: Hugh Ford
Editor: Nicola Young
Food Editor: Grace Campbell
Designer and illustrator: Sarah Odgers
Cover photography: Steve Brown
Cover stylist: Sarah O'Brien
Production Manager: Mary Bjelobrk/Alex Gonzalez

Text © Lee Holmes 2016
The moral rights of the author have been asserted.
Design © Murdoch Books 2016
Photography © Steve Brown 2016

All rights reserved. No part of this publication
may be reproduced, stored in a retrieval system or
transmitted in any form or by any means, electronic,
mechanical, photocopying, recording or otherwise,
without the prior written permission of the publisher.

A cataloguing-in-publication entry is available
from the catalogue of the National Library of
Australia at nla.gov.au.

ISBN 978 1 74336 721 6 Australia
ISBN 978 1 74336 778 0 UK

A catalogue record for this book is available from
the British Library.

Colour reproduction by Splitting Image Colour Studio
Pty Ltd, Clayton, Victoria
Printed by Hang Tai Printing Company Limited, China

IMPORTANT: Those who might
be at risk from the effects of
salmonella poisoning (the elderly,
pregnant women, young children
and those suffering from immune
deficiency diseases) should consult
their doctor with any concerns
about eating raw eggs.

OVEN GUIDE: You may find cooking
times vary depending on the oven
you are using. For fan-forced ovens,
as a general rule, set the oven
temperature to 20°C (35°F) lower
than indicated in the recipe.

MEASURES GUIDE: We
have used 20 ml (4 teaspoon)
tablespoon measures. If you
are using a 15 ml (3 teaspoon)
tablespoon add an extra teaspoon
of the ingredient for each
tablespoon specified.

DISCLAIMER: This book is
designed to provide general dietary
information for children aged six to
twelve years. The author is not
a medical professional, and the
information contained within this
book is not intended to replace
medical advice or to be relied upon
to treat, cure, or prevent any disease,
illness, or medical condition. The
author and publisher claim no
responsibility to any person or entity
for any liability, loss, or damage
caused or alleged to be caused
directly or indirectly as a result of
the use, application, or interpretation
of the material in this book.